TESTIMONIALS

"I thought I'd tried everything—and then I found this book. After years of chronic pain and weight gain and trying one prescription medicine or fad diet after another, Dr. Vickery's program changed everything. Suddenly I understood what was wrong and how to fix it—with this program for eating better, managing stress, moving my body, and finally sleeping well at night. I strongly recommend his book!"

———

"This is powerful stuff. Right now, you might not think that a positive mindset or stress management has anything to do with your health issues—but they do. Read this book. It will change how you care for yourself and, most importantly, how you feel each and every day."

———

"A smart and effective guide for living long, living healthy, and living with purpose."

———

"I spent years trying to eat healthy, but I was always coming across confusing or conflicting information. This book lays it all out there: which foods to cut, how to tailor your eating habits to your body's own needs, and how to maintain a healthy diet for long-term health."

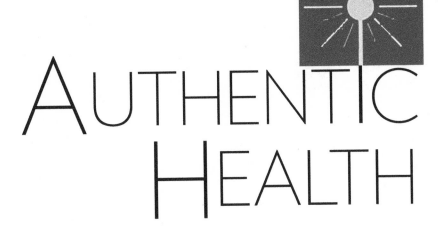

AUTHENTIC HEALTH

The Definitive Guide to Losing Weight,

Feeling Better, Mastering Stress,

Sleeping Well Every Night,

& Enjoying a Sense of Purpose

Gus Vickery, M.D.

NEW YORK

LONDON • NASHVILLE • MELBOURNE • VANCOUVER

AUTHENTIC HEALTH

The Definitive Guide to Losing Weight, Feeling Better, Mastering Stress, Sleeping Well Every Night, & Enjoying a Sense of Purpose

Published in New York, New York, by Morgan James Publishing. Morgan James is a trademark of Morgan James, LLC. www.MorganJamesPublishing.com

The Morgan James Speakers Group can bring authors to your live event. For more information or to book an event visit The Morgan James Speakers Group at www.TheMorganJamesSpeakersGroup.com.

ISBN 9781683506539 paperback
ISBN 9781683506546 eBook
Library of Congress Control Number: 2017910178

Cover Design by:
Rachel Lopez

Interior Design by:
Glen Edelstein, Hudson Valley Book Design

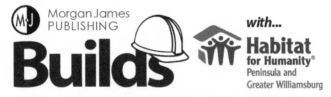

In an effort to support local communities, raise awareness and funds, Morgan James Publishing donates a percentage of all book sales for the life of each book to Habitat for Humanity Peninsula and Greater Williamsburg.

Get involved today! Visit
www.MorganJamesBuilds.com

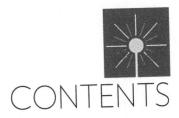

CONTENTS

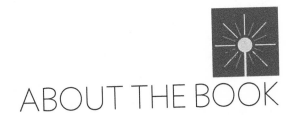

ABOUT THE BOOK

MILLIONS OF AMERICANS battle chronic physical pain, fatigue, weight gain, and persistent anxiety and depression—but when they seek help from the larger healthcare system, the only treatment available is often aimed at temporarily alleviating their symptoms rather than addressing the underlying problems. If that sounds familiar, this book is for you.

In this straightforward, easy-to-use roadmap back to health, Dr. Gus Vickery lays out a comprehensive program for addressing the habits and conditions that drive many of our painful chronic conditions. From nutrition and physical activity to lesser-known but powerfully effective techniques for managing stress, sleeping well, and cultivating a sense of purpose, Dr. Vickery offers a potent manifesto for claiming the good health that's within you.

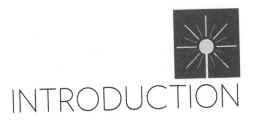

INTRODUCTION

THIS BOOK IS WRITTEN for my patients. It is also for my family, my friends, my team members within our organization, my community, and for anyone else who might find the message helpful. The information I hope to communicate is a synthesis of almost twenty years of study, personal reflection, and consultations with individuals in a medical setting.

I am a primary care physician, and I love what I do. If I had to start all over again, I would choose to be right where I am, doing what I'm doing. Each day when I go to work, I am committed to helping each of my patients find the best possible health and vitality.

The actual practice of medicine is very different from what I visualized on the day I was admitted to medical school. I was a somewhat nontraditional student. I had spent a number of years working and traveling before I decided to finish my undergraduate degree. When I went back to college in my early twenties, I studied science because I thought it was interesting. I actually expected that I would get a graduate degree and perhaps become a teacher.

When the doors opened to medical school, I was excited about the opportunity. I pictured being truly useful to others. I knew I wanted to be a general practitioner, and I had the storybook image of that in my mind. I pictured myself treating families for illness and injury, splinting fractures and sewing up lacerations. I pictured myself as a consultant to help people when life broke them in some way.

I had no idea that I would spend most of my time immersed in a quagmire of chronic diseases whose recommended treatments were often primarily supported from research funded by pharmaceutical companies.

In medical school, I studied all types of diseases and their treatments. When I learned about type 2 diabetes, for instance, I was instructed in the medications used to control it, but I don't recall any emphasis on how eating habits and lack of physical movement could significantly influence the development of the disease. As it turns out, a lot of what I learned in medical school about nutrition came from research funded by the sugar industry. Meanwhile, the research about treatments was financed by the pharmaceutical industry. I didn't understand any of this until much later in my career.

Currently, the incidence of type 2 diabetes mellitus and insulin resistance in this country is rising at disturbing rates. Since I was in medical school, there have been regularly updated "best practices" for the management of these conditions—and yet, if these were truly best practices, I firmly believe that we would have seen a reduction in the number of people afflicted, similar to what was accomplished with infectious diseases through the development of public health initiatives, vaccines and antibiotics. But we've seen nothing of the kind.

Over the same time period, the cost of healthcare has skyrocketed. As an attempt to contain costs, increasing numbers of bureaucrats entered the exam room with me. The bureaucrats felt that the best way to control the cost of healthcare was to micromanage my decisions and have me report loads of data about my patients. Suddenly, a significant percentage of the time I spent with my patients was diverted to data entry. This had little to do with the actual reasons my patients were seeking medical attention, and it disrupted the chance for deeper engagement between doctor and patient.

On top of that, standard insurance plans stopped covering the newest available medications for the treatment of chronic conditions. While it's certainly reasonable to scrutinize expensive pharmaceuticals, it's unreasonable to withhold medication and simultaneously *not* invest in the resources that would actually equip these individuals to reverse their conditions.

And so my patients with chronic conditions began to find themselves out of options. Their existing health plans were already eating up all the money they could spend on their health, and the latest treatments were no longer covered or affordable. They had very little access to the information that would help them make meaningful lifestyle changes. There was no way for me to tolerate this state of affairs; I *had* to find another way.

And we did find another way. At my medical practice, we found another way because we were committed to helping our patients find the good health within them.

We began to provide the resources necessary for our patients to change their approach to eating and reverse their chronic diseases. Soon I realized that the extra fat my patients had accumulated was not the primary issue: the underlying *habits* were creating the extra fat. And the more I dug into the habits, the more I came across information about how our food policies and treatment recommendations were influenced by for-profit companies. I also learned about how our modern technologies affect our brains. I became disturbed—and then angry—at the way individual human beings are intentionally manipulated for the purposes of creating wealth for a subset of our population.

The subtle influences were evident in the commercials that ran during the 2016 Summer Olympic Games. We rarely turn on the television in my house, but I wanted my kids to see Michael Phelps swim his final Olympic races. A single commercial break summed up what our marketing culture intends for us.

The first commercial, for a well-known soft drink, contained all kinds of imagery to suggest that this sugary drink would amplify our experiences of pleasure. The next commercial was for a telecommunications company and suggested that its data plan would lead to the social enrichment that all of us deeply desire. The next advertisement was for a cable company, and once again, there were powerful images now suggesting that our lives would be more vibrant if only we were connected to its 300 channels anywhere we go. The fourth commercial, for an insurance company, indicated that the company could protect our most precious moments in life, which we know is not true. The grand finale was a commercial for a large bank that suggested that it would help us fund all of our consumer desires.

Basically, this series of ads used powerful and emotionally evocative imagery to suggest that we should drink a soda, plug into our electronic devices, and experience the world from our couches while watching television. We also should insure these so-called comforts so that we can't lose them and pay for all of it with corporate banking.

Is this the life we want? The marketers believe that it is, and the rest of us have, unfortunately, been asleep. It's time for us to wake up and pursue our health and vitality. Our world needs individuals who are serious about their health and their purpose. We've got to reject fake foods that have been engineered to be habit-forming, turn away from the entertainment that saps our energy, and stop trusting that pharmaceuticals will bail us out of the consequences of all this fake food and addictive entertainment.

Please forgive me if I sound as if I'm ranting. I am passionate about health. I try never to judge my individual patients because of their struggles. However, I do judge how some of our systems will seductively market goods and services that have the ability to take our good health from us. I have a data plan. I watched the Olympics on cable. I use a bank and also have insurance. I am not trying to suggest that these services are all bad all of the time. I just want to enhance our awareness of how our choices are being influenced and the consequences this may have on our health.

When I began the research that ultimately led to this book, the first principle that I really dug into was how our nutritional habits were the possible cause of many of our chronic conditions. The more I looked into the history of our food sources, the more the ongoing debates about the health impact of industrialized foods puzzled me. Certain facts are overwhelmingly clear: our population is much fatter and sicker now than we were before we started consuming processed foods, and we're getting sicker all the time. You can let industrial food scientists give you lengthy, complex arguments to suggest that their products aren't the problem—or you can open your eyes and decide for yourself what is true.

Our new normal size includes an extra twenty or thirty pounds on our bodies. The extra visceral fat that we have allowed to accumulate over the past decades is a disease; it's almost like a cancer. It grows slowly and to its own advantage, while it harms the rest of our bodies. It contributes to cardiovascular disease, cancer, metabolic diseases, chronic inflammatory diseases, and a host of energy-draining conditions. If you carry this extra weight, you should want it gone from your body in any way possible. In fact, this fatty tissue, which is a consequence of chronic hormonal stimulation, actually begins to exert control of our habits due to its own hormonal influence. It is now doing this to our children.

The more I learned about the underlying causes of our poor health, the more I discussed the issues with my patients. And the more we talked, the more I understood that people truly want to be well. When given the opportunity by trusted medical professionals who genuinely care about their well-being, they are open to changing their habits in order to transform their health. In fact, for the most part, they have been trying to follow the recommendations we have provided them. It just turned out that many of our recommendations were founded on wrong assumptions about what was causing obesity and its related chronic diseases.

What you'll find in the core of this book—which covers sleep, stress,, nutrition, and physical activity—is a guidebook for changing *your* habits to transform *your* health. You just have to know the truth about which habits will take you on the journey to your best health. The approach outlined in this book is not new, and it is not a secret. It makes perfect sense when you step back from the maelstrom of information overload and just think about how our bodies and minds are designed to function.

As I wrote this book, I often felt embarrassed. It didn't seem as though we should need a book about the healthy habits that my grandparents took for granted. Not only that, but as I reviewed a substantial amount of source material, I realized that all of this information has already been published. My message is not unique. There are many individuals and entities out there talking about the same things—so who was *I* to think that *my* message should be published?

But people haven't been getting the message. Our current state of health has made me feel it is necessary, even urgent, to make this information available to my patients and to anyone else who wants it.

Indeed, we cannot wait on the current group of public health officials, insurance companies, and powerful health conglomerates to help us find our way back to health. The companies that sell us stuff will be happy to continue taking our money in exchange for our checked-out lives of television, social media, and bad food. We can't wait on these powerful interests to make the changes that we need; we have to claim our health for ourselves. If not for ourselves, then at least for our children.

Let me propose something that may sound a bit ridiculous to many people. I would suggest that, if you currently find yourself sick, overweight or obese, suffering from chronic diseases, or battling destructive habits that you just cannot seem to conquer, that it is probably not really your fault. Yes, I said it is not your fault.

Your current state of health has been largely influenced by the messages your body has been receiving. These messages come in the form of nutrition, stress, sleep, movement, and your environment. Your body and mind started receiving these messages before you took your first breath in this world. From the time you were born, you have been conditioned into behaviors and habits that significantly influence your health. Even if your parents were doing the best they could to protect your health, they were often working off of flawed information.

Perhaps you were conditioned to always eat breakfast, and that breakfast primarily contained sugary foods labeled as healthy. Perhaps you were taught to snack on processed foods between meals. Before you were old enough to make your own decisions, you were being conditioned to desire minimally nutritious, sugary foods. Also, the frequency with which you were encouraged to eat them was initiating hormonal responses within your body that begin to increase your risk of obesity. Meanwhile, if you recognized this and wanted to do something about it, the recommendations provided by public policy makers, healthcare officials, and food manufacturers actually encouraged the very same approach to nutrition that was creating the problem in the first place. You were moving further from the truth about how to be healthy even as you attempted to become healthier. When it was not working, you were told that you probably were not really doing what you were supposed to. *You* were at fault.

So you tried harder. You cut the fat out of your diet like they suggested and replaced it with healthy carbohydrates like wheat, corn, and juice. You moved more. You ate six meals a day and never missed breakfast. You gained more weight. You were told you were not following the program. You became ashamed. Finally you just decided to eat barely anything every day. You finally lost a little weight. It worked! You lost weight and felt better. For a little while. And then the weight came back no matter what you tried. Everyone figured you lacked self-control and could not follow the plan. At some point you just agreed with them and stopped trying.

Now your internal hormonal signaling has changed how it manages your appetite and energy expenditure. You eat more and move less. Everyone knew that it was all your fault all along. You agree with them as you really cannot control your appetite. No one told you that it was being driven by hormones and was not subject to your control. No one understood that your weight caused you to eat more. It was not overeating that caused you to become obese. You became obese following the advice of those who taught you how to eat.

Your eating behaviors were conditioned responses. Once you were old enough to make your own choices, you were given bad advice. Your body's own internal signaling took over the regulation of your appetite and your movement. The control center of your body, your mind, was too riddled with shame, guilt, doubt, and self-loathing to help you find your way out of the whole mess. Those offering you the solutions to this problem provided programs that were ineffective to address the underlying hormonal processes that were causing your obesity. Meanwhile, everyone pretty much blamed you for the whole thing. They figured you must just want to live with this problem. Unbelievable. Perhaps the state you find yourself in is not all your fault.

However, there is hope. There are evidence based solutions for those afflicted with these diseases. That is why I wrote this book. In order to reverse these problems you have to know the truth about your health. You have to know the truth about what causes obesity, type 2 diabetes, and other chronic diseases. If you are not provided the truth, how can you make a different choice? You will just be guessing, and the current marketplace is waiting to cash in on your efforts. You do not have to guess.

There is a truth about the ways our bodies are designed. There is a truth about the path of authentic health. This approach is not new, it is age old and time tested. It makes sense. This truth is not a secret. It is just hard to find given the information overload of our current age, and the many conflicts of interest influencing that information. I am going to provide you the truth about health. Your job is being open to making choices consistent with this truth. Once you know the truth, you have to make a choice. It does not matter whose fault it was. It is your future and your life. You have to choose- avoid change and stay sick or courageously start your journey of authentic health? You must choose. No one else can choose for you.

Your doctor cannot give you back your health. Neither can your family or your employer. You must want it for yourself. As I undertook this quest to understand authentic health better, I realized that I could only help those who truly want to be well. If a patient only wants medications and remains unwilling to change his or her lifestyle, there isn't much I can do.

I am frequently asked for my thoughts on the difference between the people who succeed in their quest for good health versus those who do not. In my opinion, the number-one factor is desire. Those who truly desire health will be willing to do whatever it takes. After that, the second greatest factor is resilience—because change is difficult. Every change involves giving something up, whether it's longstanding beliefs, habits that used to satisfy, family culture, or something else. It takes courage to give up those old habits—so you must be resilient.

I understand that you might believe that your habits are "just who you are." I mean no offense, but that's simply not true. You have the potential to be many different selves. Throughout this book we'll mention the concept of "epigenetics," which means that your DNA expresses itself at any given moment based on your environment, the people around you, your mindset (whether positive or negative), your nutrition, your movement, your sleep, and many other factors.

In other words, you have the ability to foster a healthier version of yourself, and your genetic code is standing by, waiting to help. What's more, your brain has an incredible amount of plasticity; it has the ability to overcome great trauma and to build new neural networks that will support you on your quest for health. We'll get into the details in the pages ahead, but for now, simply know that you have amazing potential within you.

When you think about the people who have qualities you admire—such as courage, integrity, discipline, self-control, and fortitude—consider that they have simply conditioned those qualities into their being. Doing so may be easier for some than others—because of factors like environment, parenting, or mentoring—but having those qualities is possible for all of us.

Imagine, for instance, that you came to me because you're sick, and I got back to you with your test results and said, "I have good news and bad news. You have a chronic disease that medical science has no cure for. The treatments we have might slow its pace, but this disease will eventually kill you—and you'll feel awful until it does. It may take decades, but it's going to happen.

"But the good news is that the disease can be reversed through a specific program of healthy nutrition, regular exercise, getting eight hours of sleep each night, and closely guarding your mind from fear-provoking stimuli. If you do these things, the disease will reverse course, and it's unlikely that it will ever harm you."

My guess is that you—and most everyone—would follow those guidelines.

That's why we must begin to think about our chronic conditions in a new way. We have to reinterpret our circumstances to understand the root causes and to initiate our desire to be well.

I believe we all have the ability to become our best selves. Your brain is incredibly powerful, and you have the power to interpret your circumstances as a positive part of your story.

The process itself is important. The journey toward good health is where you write your own story, on your own terms. I'll give you some basics in this book, but it will be up to you to identify the deeper purpose that motivates you to choose health. Meanwhile, the universe stands ready to align its forces behind those who have the courage to pursue their best selves and create a better future.

How does this look in real life? Let's consider two different individuals, both named Mary. Both Marys grew up in similar circumstances. They both experienced many good things in their lives, including meaningful relationships, a fairly long lifespan with mostly stable health, and the opportunity to engage in meaningful work interspersed with restful vacations. They also had negative experiences. Both of them had been hurt by others, and both had experienced frustrating and disappointing circumstances and dealt with periods of physical and emotional pain associated with injury or illness.

Now, at age 80, they are both dying from metastatic cancer in a hospice facility. Neither of them will live more than a few weeks. They are both cared for by a team of compassionate medical professionals. Family and friends visit them both regularly. One of these Marys feels very loved and cared for. She feels she had a blessed life, full of meaning. She is grateful, courageous, peaceful, and comfortable. She sees the beauty and goodness in those caring for her and in those visiting her. Although her cancer is causing her pain, this does not seem to negatively impact her interpretation of her circumstances. She is at peace, and that is her reality.

The other Mary feels victimized by her cancer and pain. She feels angry that she is no longer in her own home and in control of her circumstances. She feels her family has betrayed her by arranging for her to be in the hospice facility. She remembers the times she was wronged throughout her life and feels that she was never given the opportunity to live the life she deserved. This Mary is in pain, and the medications do not seem to help. This Mary feels lonely despite the visits from her family. This Mary is fearful, depressed, and angry. This is her interpretation of her circumstances, and it is her reality.

These two Marys have identical circumstances and very similar histories. But now they are experiencing two very different realities—solely because of how their minds are narrating their stories.

There's nothing unusual about their stories. In my medical practice I have been continually amazed by my patients' ability to overcome terrible afflictions. I have seen people who have every right to complain, but they choose, instead, to express only gratitude. I have also seen people who live privileged lives with minimal discomfort who complain unceasingly. It has become clear to me that each person's vitality is closely related to his or her mindset.

The fact that you've picked up this book suggests that you're ready to take control of your health. In the pages ahead, we will focus on the importance of your thinking and mindset. We will discuss the concept of purpose as a foundation for building a healthy and rewarding life.

Then we will move into the doing. We will discuss a practical and accessible approach to using meditation and breath control for improving your focus and awareness and reducing your stress responses. We will provide a concise overview of how to source your food in a healthy way and outline an approach to eating that can help initiate and *sustain* weight loss. We will train you in how to become an expert sleeper, and we will help you develop a habit of physical movement that will invigorate your body and give you energy. The result will be a healthier you.

Through all of this, it is important to understand that there is no specific arrival point on this journey. Once started, you are embarking on an ongoing quest. Until the day you die, you will still be thinking about how to have a healthier mind and body. You will still be thinking about how to be fully alive in every present moment and how to interpret these moments in the most positive way possible.

Please keep in mind that this book is meant to be a concise summary of each of the core areas that drive your health. It's not meant to be an exhaustive scientific text or a comprehensive guide to the solutions. I've included sufficient action steps and information for you to integrate this content into your daily life without further study—but I would encourage you to dive more deeply into the concepts described here. To that end, I have included a list of additional materials for each area of discussion that can take you further into the concepts and enrich your understanding.

However, I encourage you to keep things very simple. The best way to make progress towards a goal is to focus on one thing at a time. Do this one thing until it becomes your new habit and then pick the next thing. My list of additional resources is purposely brief. I have provided more comprehensive lists of additional resources at our web based resource hub www.healthshepherds.com.

As I wrote this book, I was tempted to make it longer and more comprehensive. My doctor's brain wanted to make this book impressive to my colleagues and those who write books on complex topics. I wanted to use citations and data tables and support my opinions with lengthy scientific explanations. However, my patients helped me to understand what they desired. They wanted me to keep this simple. I wrote this book for my patients and anyone else whose life could improve with this information. For those who want more comprehensive data and citations, please review the additional resources I reference. My purpose in this book is to be an effective translator of this information. My goal is to inspire everyone to desire their best health.

While this book may come across as lengthy to some, I want to emphasize how simple and natural good health can be. Our bodies are designed well. We are designed to be healthy and have energy. Chronic diseases are not normal, especially in our children. Your good health does not require lengthy lists of do's and don'ts. All you need to do is to be intentional about a few key habits and your good health will be manifested.

We have to help each other with this. We have to stop blaming ourselves and others and start helping each other become our healthiest selves. This is not just about our individual good health. This is about creating a new conversation about authentic health for all people everywhere.

I sincerely hope this message helps you. It has certainly helped me.

Gus Vickery, MD
www.healthshepherds.com

HOW TO USE THIS BOOK

WHILE EACH CHAPTER of this book can serve as a stand-alone resource on its given topic, the flow of the book is intentional. The first chapters offer practical steps for building a strong desire for genuine health, as well as for building the mindset to achieve it. The second half of the book addresses nutrition, mastering stress, movement, and sleep. At the end of each of these chapters, you'll find a section called "Step into the consultation room." This simulates how I would integrate the chapter's material into an action plan if you were my patient. Each "Step into the consultation room" section builds on the section from the previous chapter, while also integrating the new. They also provide action steps to begin to build these practices into your own life. I encourage you to get started with these steps, or with any other changes you are able to make, no matter how small. Any positive change at all will initiate responses in you that increase the likelihood of further positive change. Just start. Pick something, and do it. Meditate for three minutes, or write down your health goals. Pick one healthier food, and take a ten-minute walk. Just *start*. If you follow the suggestions in this book, you *will* become healthier.

At the very end of each chapter, you'll find a list of resources that will teach you more about the core content of each chapter, if you wish to go deeper.

Some of the content is in the form of photographs, videos, and PDF documents which can all be viewed or downloaded at our web resource hub- www.healthshepherds.com.

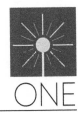

ONE

There's No Law That Says You Have To Be Sick

YOUR BODY *HURTS*.

Your muscles and joints ache and there's pain in your chest and stomach. Your mind is foggy; you have trouble concentrating. You get headaches and you just don't have energy the way you used to. It's affecting your mood, too. You feel down a lot of the time—and that's making it hard to sleep.

Eventually you think to yourself, "I've got to go see somebody." You know all these health problems might get in the way of your job if they keep getting worse.

So you go see your doctor.

She identifies a few issues. There are some problems with your posture and some muscle weakness. She has concerns about your nutrition. She says you need to make changes to your diet and lose some weight.

It sounds daunting. "How am I going to do that?" you ask.

She says that, ideally, you'd work with a physical therapist on core strength and muscle lengthening, and maybe also a "medical manual therapist"—someone like a masseuse. She says you'd also benefit from seeing an expert nutritionist and possibly a counselor to help with your mood. In fact, she'd really like to get you in to see an engaging counseling specialist who could help you develop some habits around positive thinking to address your chronic melancholy. Counseling would not only improve your mood, but it would help you concentrate during the day and then sleep soundly at night.

It all sounds—expensive. "Is my insurance going to cover that?" you ask.

No. Most services aren't covered, and those that are carry $75 co-pays because they're considered specialties. You would need to go twice a week. There's no way you can afford that. It's off the table.

But your doctor wants to help you as best she can. She orders a few tests to make sure there's nothing more serious going on that she missed in her examination. Then she prescribes a muscle relaxer and an anti-inflammatory to ease your physical discomfort. She also gets you on an antidepressant.

You feel better—for a while.

But soon, you realize you feel exactly the same as before, only now you're on a slew of medications. Meanwhile, the anti-inflammatory could give you a stomach ulcer, and the muscle relaxer could get you into a car accident because it's a sedative. And you're going to need to keep switching from one antidepressant to another, since the effect of each one just seems to kind of … peter out.

All of this is expensive, too. It's not as pricey as seeing specialists, but the prescription co-pays add up. All the doctor visits and medications will probably drive up the cost of your insurance coverage next year, though you might not personally see that cost if your insurance is covered by your employer. Far worse, you may be headed for much bigger medical bills around the corner, because your health is still declining.

You're stuck in this rut. With each thing you try, you end up coming back to the same poor health. You're physically and emotionally exhausted.

But there's another way.

This book is about finding your health in the only place it can truly be found: within you. This book is about the simple and truthful approaches that will allow you to experience authentic health—which is your birthright.

Many people are chronically sick in ways that are complicated and are related to their habits and behaviors—and yet they don't realize it. We all have our individual habits, of course. Those habits determine how we start the day, how much coffee we drink, which foods we choose, how we sit at our desks or hold our bodies all day long, how we breathe, what we drink, how we manage stress, how we play, how we distract ourselves to escape from the things that feel burdensome, how we manage our relationships with others, and how we prepare ourselves to sleep at night and do it all again tomorrow.

Though many of us never give much thought to these sorts of habits, together they add up to how much mental, physical, and emotional energy each of us has to put toward our life's purpose.

What's more, our behaviors tend to be heavily influenced by savvy companies that have something to sell us. They sell us cheap and tasty food. They sell us digital entertainment that keeps us parked in our chairs or absorbed in our phones. They also sell us the pharmaceuticals that are supposed to make us feel better when all the cheap food and digital entertainment have taken a toll on our bodies.

What's more, these companies are intimately involved in the nonprofit organizations and governmental agencies that are supposed to set health standards and look out for our best interests. A recent study by two health researchers found that two major soda companies make donations—often in the millions of dollars—to the most influential health foundations and government health institutes, and they often succeed at buying influence over our national "health" agenda.[1]

The upshot of all these factors is an astonishing incidence of chronic illness across the country. Arthritis, chronic fatigue, muscle pain, depression, anxiety, obesity, and insomnia—to name just a few—are sapping our energy and our potential. We are plagued by the metabolic diseases that accompany obesity such as diabetes, high blood pressure, and arterial disease. There are autoimmune conditions. There are cancers. There is also brain fog and short-term memory loss. Patients who are only 45 years old come to see me and ask, "Could I already have dementia?" They're losing their ability to concentrate.

But there's no law that says you have to be sick. And in this book, you'll find a powerful alternative. This alternative is not new, and it isn't a fad that will be released in much-hyped installments over a period of several weeks. On the contrary, it's the age-old, time-tested formula for human beings to be well.

In truth, we shouldn't have to search for the secrets to health or read about them in a book. But in the 21st century, we *do* have to search—be-

---

1   Daniel G. Aaron and Michael B. Siegel, "Sponsorship of National Health Organizations by Two Major Soda Companies," *American Journal of Preventive Medicine* (2016).

cause our ability to see what drives our own health has been so obscured by the deceptive marketing of vast corporations whose sole purpose is to make more money. What should be self-evident has become hidden behind cheap products that are purposely designed to be habit-forming and that keep us overweight, exhausted, unfulfilled, and potentially very sick.

We must not put up with this unfortunate state of affairs for even one more second.

Meanwhile, at your local doctor's office, you would ideally have access to the resources you need to get healthy again. But however skilled and dedicated your doctor is, he or she is constrained by a tangle of rules that are largely set by insurance companies. In other words, in addition to facing a mass of corporations that profit from making you sick—and even as you or your employer or the government pay a hefty amount of money for your health insurance—we *also* have a "health" system that is designed to keep you from being well.

A HEALTHCARE SYSTEM THAT'S FAILING TO CARE FOR OUR HEALTH

As I'll explain in detail later, your health is the sum of your habits. Companies selling you unhealthy products have likely influenced your habits and thereby caused or contributed to your painful, chronic conditions. On top of that, we have a healthcare "system" that is really just a sprawling and disjointed assembly of health companies and programs—and it's doing nothing to reverse this trend.

Maybe you're struggling with headaches and fatigue and bloating and reflux. Maybe you find that your joints ache after you eat. So you go on the Internet and enter your symptoms. A host of medical diagnoses pop up, including things like "tension headaches." The website says a few things about the cause of your symptoms, but it can't give you all you need to know about your problem.

We have a health system that treats symptoms instead of conditions. Your search might have turned up a few resources about lack of sleep, or about diet, or about stress management, or lack of exercise, but there's too much conflicting information.

Patients come into my office all the time and tell me that their bodies hurt after they eat. Sometimes they come in because they've seen a commercial advertising a medicine to deal with precisely this problem. As a doctor, I've got to do some due diligence; I ask about their habits and about what they're eating. "What did you eat before you experienced these symptoms?" I ask. Often, the answer is a chilidog and a soda, or something similar.

The pain and reflux and heartburn and general discomfort that follow after we eat our favorite foods are *symptoms*. And in our existing health system, we tend to ask, "What can I do about these symptoms?

But we don't ask the underlying question: "What condition is *causing* these symptoms?"

There are pills to treat your symptoms, of course. But those pills are little more than a Band-Aid. They're a temporary solution. And even as they're providing temporary relief, they create new problems that will also, in turn, need solutions.

When your body hurts—whether it's a headache, or heartburn, or fatigue, or aches in your joints—your body is telling you something. In fact, your body is sending you an important message that something you're doing isn't working. Some of your habits are causing harm. The pain is a symptom; the underlying *habit* is what's driving the problem.

You're not alone. Statistics overwhelmingly show that we've become a less healthy population. Meanwhile the health infrastructure that's supposed to make us healthy is, instead, stuck on treating our symptoms instead of their causes.

In our current system, you see a medical professional either because you're experiencing symptoms or because you're having a routine checkup. In the first case, the appointment tends to revolve explicitly around treating those symptoms, and you'll walk out the door with a new prescription. In the second case, the practitioner examines you based on guidelines and algorithms passed down from the Department of Health and Human Services. If you're twenty-five, that means the doctor is going to counsel you about not texting and driving, plus the dangers of syphilis. In other words, when you go into a healthcare office, generally the agenda isn't about your specific situation—it's about the priorities of the larger system.

But obviously, that's not going to move the needle on your individual health. When you come in for your checkup, the public-health priorities ("don't text and drive" or "don't have unprotected intercourse") are quickly completed. It's straightforward. And that's the entire agenda.

An assessment of your real health, and your underlying habits, isn't part of the deal. What's more, physicians' offices have to spend so much time on coding and billing the insurance companies that there's not enough time left over to probe the more complicated stuff. You might be cognitively depressed and physically exhausted. You might be sleeping poorly and losing energy. It's unlikely that a routine check-up will result in real solutions to address these significant underlying problems.

It's not the fault of the medical practitioners at that office—far from it. Let's say you mention that you're struggling with depression and that you're having trouble sleeping. Maybe the doctor is well aware that you'd benefit from cognitive behavioral therapy. But helping you get that therapy is not that simple.

Until very recently, your insurance likely wouldn't have covered any sort of mental-health care at all. Recent changes in health care have increased the likelihood that mental-health services are covered equally with other types of care; that's a good thing, because we should make sure that the brain isn't treated as some separate thing from the body. But even so, those behavioral health services are going to cost you. You'll probably face a high deductible. Not to mention that you've got to drive someplace every week and spend an hour of your time with a therapist. In other words, getting this treatment is not straightforward.

The same goes for nutrition. Maybe your diet is contributing to chronic diseases and potentially causing serious long-term damage to your health. In that case, it's important for you really to begin to understand what different types of food do to your body. Maybe you *want* to change your habits. A nutritionist would be a great resource. But it turns out that the nutritionist is expensive and that you're going to run into the same problem with the high deductible.

So even in the best-case scenario, with a physician who really wants to help you change your habits, none of the necessary interventions seem accessible. And thus, in all likelihood, you're going to continue with the same habits you've always had.

This book is about giving you options. It's about giving you control over your health. It's about not settling for poor health because of an inadequate healthcare system. You do *not* have to remain stuck in chronic illness. With intentionality, you can create the right habits and behaviors.

You can choose health.

GUARDING A CORE PURPOSE—YOURS, AND MINE

My philosophy is grounded in the belief that every individual has a dignified purpose. If all of us can find a way to manifest that purpose, then we will flourish. Everyone has that potential.

I also believe that it's our job as a society to create systems that help every person flourish. Right now, we're falling pretty short of that goal because we have economic and health systems that make it difficult for us to access the good health within us.

That's why this book is written to you as an individual. Our larger system isn't working. You're the only one who can make this change for you.

I've come to this conclusion after more than a decade practicing as a primary-care physician. My passion is to help people truly become healthy. Early on in my practice, I realized that the factors that influenced my patients' health were complex, and that many of the prevailing treatment strategies were superficial. The more I dug into the root causes of diseases that manifested as symptoms, the more I began to recognize the significance of habits and behaviors.

Over the years, I pored through the biomedical literature as well as research in the fields of nutrition, cognitive behavioral therapy, and physical activity. At the same time, I was also spending five days a week seeing my patients, which is a continual source of learning for me. Every encounter in the exam room teaches me something: What *actually* works? Which interventions make the most sense for which circumstances?

The philosophy in this book is the distillation of all those years of studying and probing—and in these pages you'll find a formula for good health.

You will *not* find recommendations for specific fads. I won't be telling you, for instance, that the latest and greatest fitness or nutrition program is the answer for you. Instead, you'll find a more fundamental, evidence-based, time-tested guide for claiming and improving your own health. If that's what you're seeking, then this book is for you.

I believe every individual has a dignified purpose—and that this is mine. I chose primary care because I wanted to work one-on-one with my patients and care for their whole health. My passion for this work is what sent me to seek better solutions to my patients' ailments. It's what sent me into the annals of medical literature to grapple with the best science out there in order to get to the root causes of poor health. And that led me to the philosophy that's in this book.

I'm also the father of three children whom I love very much. As a parent, I wanted to know how to raise children who will be able to intentionally *choose* their habits—rather than having those habits chosen for them—so that they can show up to life with the greatest possible energy and potential. That, too, is part of my core purpose, and it has motivated the development of the philosophy that you'll find in these pages.

I have colleagues who think I'm crazy for going into primary care in such a challenging time. That doesn't bother me; I'm doing what I'm meant to be doing. I know because my patients tell me how much I've helped them. There are people who've been with me for many years who tell me that their lives are better because of the work that I did with them. That affirms my core purpose more than any paycheck or collegial respect ever could.

It's not an easy time to be a doctor, of course. The insurance companies try to pay me less for the same work. They may try to coerce me into providing care according to their specific rules. But nobody can take from me my core purpose, which is to help every patient find the best health they can. Once a patient enters into a confidential consult in our examining room, we focus on *their* needs. Of course, I have to fulfill my obligations to the insurance companies and bureaucrats, but once I've done that, we can focus on how to care for *this* individual.

And this book is the same; it's about helping you to actualize *your* purpose, and to do so by giving you back your health.

IT'S EASIER THAN YOU THINK

In the next chapters, you're going to read some inspiring stories about how individuals like you began to modify their behaviors and habits and eventually created a new story about their health—and, in turn, about their lives.

Before we get to that, though, it's important to acknowledge that such change can be intimidating. You might not be sure that you're up for it, and I can understand that. Our habits are our habits for a reason. We eat the foods we eat because they taste good. We engage in the behaviors we do because they're how we've always done things. There are only so many hours in the day—and so much energy in your bones—to try new things.

But consider this. It's possible that never, for a single day in your life, have you felt the depth of energy that you actually possess inside of you. It's possible that you have never once felt as good as you're capable of feeling.

If you're willing to take a chance on a few low-risk strategies that you agree would be good for your health, then you may be taking the first step toward a level of physical vitality and mental clarity that will astonish you. And it may well impress you so much that you'll never want to return to your old habits again.

If you're willing to consider that you may be missing out on something incredible, read on.

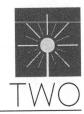

TWO

I'm Writing This Book Because I Want You To Feel Better

THERE'S A TROUBLING difference between what they teach aspiring doctors in medical school and what happens in the actual, everyday practice of medicine.

In medical school, I learned that health is a complicated mix of factors that go far deeper than the physical body. This even has a name in the medical parlance: it's called the *biopsychosocial* model, which just means that the roots of disease aren't only in the body but also include psychological factors—that is, your personality and your day-to-day behavior and disposition—as well as social factors, such as your family and cultural surroundings. When I was a medical student, I learned that I was supposed to take these complicated variables into account in order to diagnose and treat illness.

But after medical school, young doctors leap from the classroom to the examining room, and the time necessary for truly considering a biopsychosocial model is just not available. Doctors see dozens of patients every day. The pace and realities of modern practice don't allow for much—or any—consideration of those deeper determinants of health. Physicians only have time to deal with *symptoms*, rather than the underlying *causes* of those symptoms.

Meanwhile, the way insurance companies try to honor the biopsychosocial model is by providing lots of questionnaires for you to fill out, often before you've even met your healthcare provider, which then get scanned and added to your chart. These questionnaires are supposed to capture the important details of your family, your history, and your psychology. Of course, an impersonal questionnaire is unlikely to achieve anything like that—but if you've ever wondered why you have to fill out all that paperwork, now you know.

At the same time, requirements set by these same insurance companies effectively eat up all the time doctors could devote to really *talking* with their patients about the material in those questionnaires. That is, the one person you might trust enough to discuss such personal information with—your doctor—doesn't have nearly enough time to do so.

Let's say a doctor is seeing her twenty-second patient of the day, and it's someone who says he can't sleep. Immediately the doctor asks herself: how do we treat insomnia? Well, there's a class of medications that help insomnia. Bingo! She writes a prescription.

This doctor doesn't have time to get into the fact that the insomnia might be the result of excessive exposure to computer screens well into the evening—or the possibility that this patient is anxious and doesn't know how to settle his mind down in order to sleep, and that's why he's waking up in the middle of the night.

The doctor also doesn't have time to delve into the potential for this insomnia eventually to cause depression: A prolonged lack of sleep leads to fatigue, loss of motivation, problems with concentration and focus, and a feeling of a lack of purpose, all of which can produce depression.

On top of that, once you're depressed, your eating habits tend to change, and you often end up gaining weight—and the mix of all these different ailments will make it extremely difficult for you to lose that weight once you've put it on. But the doctor doesn't have time to get into that. So the patient will go on his way with a prescription for an insomnia medicine, but his health will only get worse.

Of course, there are some conditions that we doctors are genuinely effective at treating. People come in with broken bones. They come in needing stitches. They have infections. We do a good job on that type of stuff; there's a specific set of applicable resources for putting those people back together. Thank goodness we can help them! But those aren't the conditions I'm talking about.

What about all the people who come in because they're exhausted, because they have high blood pressure, because they're overweight, because their bodies hurt, because they have reflux? It's all the patients who have a complicated set of issues whose treatment requires much more than a few stitches or a pill. These patients require much more than a brief office visit, but the breakneck pace of modern medicine doesn't allow for that.

With this as background, you won't be surprised to know that young doctors often quickly feel overwhelmed. We get frustrated. "I can't do all this!" we say to ourselves. And we fall into the habit of doing what all the doctors before us have done: we write prescriptions. We get really good at writing prescriptions, because that's a tool we can use when we only have a few minutes per patient. Maybe we also make a few recommendations—like weight loss—but those recommendations often don't go anywhere.

"Well, how am I going to lose weight?" the patient asks.

"Well, there's Weight Watchers," we might say. Or there's this resource, or that one.

"Will my insurance cover it?" the patient asks.

For the first five years of my career, most types of insurance still had relatively affordable deductibles and copays, and they had pretty decent prescription drug coverage. However, obesity management was considered cosmetic, so there was often no coverage at all for weight-loss programs.

That's changed. Over time, our country has increasingly relied on expensive prescription drugs to treat conditions whose root causes are actually behavioral. That situation has created a need for even more (and even more expensive) pharmaceuticals. And that, in turn, has led to the situation in which we find ourselves—where insurance covers less, even though it costs more. Our entire country is going bankrupt over health costs, even as we find ourselves in continually worse health.

You could call it a perfect storm.

I wasn't long out of medical school when I realized that my work as a doctor was something very different from what I'd wanted and envisioned. I wasn't making people well. Instead, I was spending most of my time essentially putting Band-Aids on complicated problems that had deeper roots. I had sick patients who continued to get sicker. All I did was perhaps slow the rate at which they became less healthy. At the same time, my patients and their employers were spending more and more money on health insurance that didn't come even close to meeting its promise of providing access to "health" care.

That's when I asked, "What's *really* going on?"

A BETTER WAY

When I first began combing the literature to understand how to truly help my patients instead of sticking Band-Aids on their problems, I was astonished to discover that the sum total of all the medical research was one gigantic puzzle. Nobody had the single, definitive answer that I was looking for. The best of medical science couldn't even make up its mind on something as simple as calcium supplements. I realized there would be no straightforward answer to the complex questions I was asking.

Yet there *were* answers—they just weren't straightforward. There was useful material on cognitive behavioral therapies and motivational interviewing written by psychologists. There was important information on insomnia written by sleep specialists. There was good insight on biomechanical health written by experts who ranged from doctors to Navy SEALs. There were about a million useful resources on nutrition. And while I found definitive manuals for overall health that put all of this material together in one place, those books were too complicated to be useful for anyone without training in the medical sciences. That wasn't a problem so far as I was concerned, though, because now I was starting to see a comprehensive solution.

A few pieces of wisdom rose to the surface. The best information out there suggested that we take care of our bodies in a way that's in sync with how our bodies were designed. In other words, we need sleep. We need exercise. We need real—unprocessed—foods. Actually, amidst the vast jumble of research and data, it seemed apparent that the clearest driver of our worsening health over the past couple of generations had been the dramatic shift in what we eat and how often we eat. We're going to get into this topic in depth, but the bottom line is this: all the processed food leads to deeply troubling consequences.

I decided to put all of these findings into a single, comprehensive curriculum to help my patients take back control of their health. Together with my staff, we wrote a three-month weight-management plan that followed the best evidence-based standards. It was a step-by-step, bariatric program that provided all the necessary tools to replicate proven success in weight loss for patients with obesity and related issues.

That wasn't all. We also drew on findings from cognitive behavioral therapy in order to help patients change their habits *permanently*. You will understand the significance of this if you've ever lost ten pounds on a diet only to gain fifteen pounds a couple months down the road.

We created a physical health assessment designed so the patient could begin to change his or her habits in a gradual and sustainable way, and thus move permanently to a baseline of good health. We also developed a comprehensive nutritional curriculum that was an essential piece of this larger whole. As soon as these new materials were ready, we began offering them to our patients. We discovered that they couldn't *wait* to get started, because they'd been battling the same health problems for far too long.

Shortly after we began releasing this new curriculum to our patients, a coincidence of timing allowed me to see these solutions in action across an entire population. The Biltmore Company, a large business in my region of western North Carolina, partnered with my organization to oversee an onsite health clinic for its employees. This healthcare model was entirely different from the industry standard. For starters, The Biltmore Company employees could visit the clinic at no charge. On top of that, the medical team—which included me as well as an outstanding physician's assistant and one other excellent administrative professional—did not bill insurers for every office visit, test, and procedure in order to get paid. Instead, we received a set amount of money from The Biltmore Company with the mandate to care for the patient population as best we could.

That might not sound revolutionary, but modern medical practice is heavily limited by what insurance companies allow. That limitation had just disappeared. Moreover, the company management team, my medical colleagues, and I were jointly committed to the shared goal of truly improving patients' health, and to do so by using whichever interventions made the most sense, traditional or otherwise.

That meant we were suddenly able to employ treatments like motivational interviewing and one-on-one counseling about nutrition. In many ways, this little clinic was the very opposite of our larger healthcare system. All the barriers that usually stand between the patient and good health—from cost, to wait time, to rules set by insurance companies, to the typically hectic schedule of the medical staff—all had been removed.

So what happened?

We started seeing improvements much more quickly than we'd thought possible. People lost weight. They felt less stressed. They felt cared for. Diabetics with long-standing poor blood sugar control suddenly had better control, and some of them were reversing their diabetes altogether. They were sleeping better. They had more energy. They simply *felt* better. We saw people come alive.

Meanwhile, we were seeing similar results with our nutritional curriculum in our primary care practice. Soon, our diabetics were coming off their insulin. Other patients began dropping a whole host of different medications. People who used to be depressed were coming off their antidepressants. People were walking into my office saying, "I don't need my sleep apnea machine anymore. I feel great. I feel energetic, and I'm sleeping well."

Given a genuine opportunity, most people will choose to be well. Insurance companies seem to proceed on the opposite philosophy: that they somehow have to *force* people to be well.

I discovered that this new, invigorating good health was infectious. As if my patients had released pollen into the air around them, their friends and family members started calling my office to ask about our approach to health. Patients began transferring to our practice.

"I hear you can help me find new ways of doing things so I actually get healthy," people said when they called to make appointments. "I'm just sick of taking all these meds."

Finally I had *real* answers.

I was still seeing dozens of patients in brief appointments every day in my regular practice. But every time I walked into the examining room and saw a person who could benefit from this program, I did everything possible to get them moving in the right direction. Often, I had to talk faster in order to beat the clock. Since patients tend to go six months or a year between medical appointments, I felt—and feel—a huge sense of urgency to make sure every single patient knew there were choices. I didn't want anyone to lose another six months or a year to poor health.

"We can help you!" I said again and again. "Talk to my staff. Talk to our nutritionist. Let me give you the quick way of addressing sleep. I want you to know about sleep hygiene. I want you to know how to calm your mind and what happens during stress responses." In many cases, as soon as a patient heard a little of what was possible, they would light up.

"I really need this," they would say. "I know that you don't have much more time, but ..."

That was when I realized I needed to write it all down. Hence the book you're holding in your hands. I wanted to make sure that everyone who's seeking good health could find it.

GOOD HEALTH TRANSFORMED HIM

A kind, middle-aged man from Appalachia exemplifies the reversal that's possible with this comprehensive approach to health and wellness. This particular patient came to see me for severe varicose veins and edema, which is fluid retention in the legs. He also had developed a form of cellulitis, and by the time I saw him, he had a staph infection. He was very sick. He had a fever. I treated him with a long course of antibiotics to stabilize the infection.

But the infection and his varicose veins and the edema were all side effects of his primary ailment, which was obesity. His body mass index was over 40, which qualifies as severe obesity.

He felt a lot better after we got the infection under control, but he was still suffering from the swelling in his legs. He wanted to know what we could do about it.

"You can wear compression hose and elevate your legs and watch your salt intake," I said, "but really, this has to do with your weight."

At first, he didn't want to deal with his weight. But pretty soon, he was back in my office with another infection—and this second one was worse than the first. He nearly ended up in the hospital. Once again I treated the infection which briefly stabilized him. And then we were back to square one. He wanted to know what we could do about his increasingly poor health.

"Well, to be honest, it's your obesity," I said. "You do have varicose veins, and it's true that they are causing this recent problem. But it's your severe obesity that's creating the bigger problem."

I explained that if he didn't lose weight, he wouldn't be able to get the pooled blood and extra fluid out of his legs—even with surgery. I told him that it would just continue to come back, and that he would continue to get infections. Eventually, the staph would become treatment-resistant; at that point, his only option would be intravenous antibiotics. If it got really bad, he might develop open wounds. There was the potential that he would need an amputation, or that he would end up with an abscess that could kill him.

"The only real answer is to lose weight."

"How am I going to do that?"

Because of the extremity of his obesity, he was going to need a very structured nutrition plan. "I can provide you with all the tools and resources you need, but you're going to have to set your mind to it," I said. "Are you ready to do that?"

"I'm ready," he said. "I have to work. I have a life. I can't keep doing this. And my wife is worried about me."

I said I would help him visualize precisely what he wanted for himself, and that I would encourage him with regular reminders about his personal goals. But I explained that, moment to moment, it was going to be challenging, because he would have to change some deeply ingrained habits.

To help him get started, we would put him on a medication to stabilize his appetite. I told him, that, after a couple months, his body would get used to the changes and he wouldn't need that prescription any longer. My staff and I set him up with our comprehensive curriculum, and we made a plan to check in with him every week.

Fast-forward eighteen months. There were ups and downs and plateaus. But in the end, he lost more than 100 pounds.

Most people don't think it's possible to lose 100 pounds. But he was determined not to be sick. Being sick was not consistent with his view of himself and his purpose in life. So he did what had to be done. I'm deeply proud of him.

He still comes in for regular checkups, but he's not sick anymore. He still has some varicose veins and edema, but it's far better. He no longer gets infections. His legs no longer hurt. He doesn't wake up at night with pain and throbbing. His mood is better, his energy is better, and he finally sleeps well. He's also become a positive force for those around him. He's persuaded many of his friends to become healthier, too. He feels good about himself and his capabilities. His *life* is better.

Four years have passed now, and he hasn't regained those 100 pounds.

LEARNING TO BE YOUR OWN HEALTHCARE SYSTEM

Now you know that our existing health infrastructure isn't really a health "system," but rather a patchwork of many different companies and programs. Well, your first step to wellness is to begin to act as your *own* healthcare system. The coming chapters will provide all the information and resources that you need to find good health—in ways that include weight loss but also go far deeper, into the determinants of true health. The man from Appalachia succeeded because he was truly committed to getting well. Your key to success will be making your own commitment and then acting as your own health system.

Don't worry. It's easier than you think.

And before we go in-depth into such important areas as nutrition, stress management, and the science of sleep, I want you to have a cheat sheet so you know which things you'll need to focus on in order to be a healthcare system unto yourself. Basically, you're going to want to pay attention to a few major areas of your life that have big effects on your overall health.

For starters, it will mean becoming aware of your own thinking. Positive thinking is important for this process. You'll need to focus on your goals and visualize the kind of health you want for yourself—and you'll need to really believe in your ability to become healthy. Yes, you absolutely *can* become healthy! If my patient from Appalachia was able to lose 100 pounds, then you can tackle the problems facing you, too!

In order to cultivate this sort of positive thinking, you'll also need to pay attention to what you allow into your mind every day. Think about the kinds of entertainment that you watch or listen to or read on your phone or TV or tablet or anywhere else. Think about whether you're being manipulated and coerced into spending your time, money, and energy on cheap products and cheap entertainment. Then start to orient yourself toward making conscious choices that will benefit your health, including your mental health.

You're also going to want to start thinking about the way you hold your body all day each day, from the way you engage with your environment at home to work to anywhere else you're spending your time. Start noticing your posture as well as where and when your body starts to hurt. Pretty soon, you're going to make some small but important changes in how you move through your daily environment in order to improve your biomechanics, and your awareness of these details will be important.

Then, of course, there's nutrition. Being your own healthcare system means paying attention to what you're putting into your body and making sure that it's actually nutritious. When you walk down the aisles of the grocery story, there are lots of things labeled "healthy"—but many profit hungry food manufacturers are doing the labeling and, as it turns out, those items by and large *aren't* healthy. Many of the things we eat actually contribute to inflammation and disease.

Soon, you're going to learn to select foods that give you energy rather than take away your energy, and you're going to know how to select foods in a way that isn't manipulated by companies trying to get your money. Being your own healthcare system means ensuring that your nourishment serves its real purpose, which is to fuel your machine so you can show up to life with energy.

Then there's the way you sleep at night. This matters in a big way. Many of us tend to think that we really don't need much sleep and that we can function just fine on a couple of hours. Maybe you've learned to tolerate such little sleep, but eventually, it will cause your body to crash. Part of being your own healthcare system is embracing the notion that deep, restorative sleep in essential to your health. Soon, using the best wisdom from cognitive behavioral therapy, you'll learn techniques to quiet your mind and create an environment that's conducive to sleep. But for now, it's important simply to recognize that sleep is a top priority, and that you've got to do everything you can to get a full night's rest.

Finally, there's the power of stress management. You've got to be intentional about managing your emotions, or the injurious effects of stress will undo all the improvements in your health that you achieve through good nutrition, exercise, and sleep. In Chapter Six you'll learn meditation techniques and exercises for maintaining a focused and calm mind. By reducing your responses to stress, you'll feel better and be more resilient in both mind and body.

YOU'RE ON YOUR WAY TO TRANSFORMATIVE GOOD HEALTH

You've just taken your first steps on the pathway to long-term good health.

Though you might be trying to lose 20 or 50 or 100 pounds, you've just embarked on something far more profound than weight loss. These changes are the way to feel truly better—in perpetuity. Once achieved, this is a state of well-being that you'll be able to sustain with minimal effort. In fact, it won't feel like any effort at all, because you'll be so hooked on feeling good that you won't be willing to go back to the old way of doing things. And that will allow you finally to turn your focus and energy away from chronic poor health and toward your life's purpose.

Let's get started.

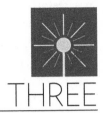

THREE

What Does It Take To Keep A Body Healthy?

This chapter provides a basic lesson in how your hormonal and metabolic systems function so that you understand why a holistic approach to your health is necessary. This chapter is a basic owner's manual for your metabolism which will help you understand how to manage your weight and your energy.

THIS BOOK IS about giving you the tools you need to be healthy. And while that might have been simple and straightforward a couple of generations ago, it's not so simple in our modern world. Our processed foods, our screens and devices, our sedentary lifestyles, and our increased chronic stress levels associated with modern life all make it difficult for us to access the good health that's within us. In this chapter and the ones that follow, you'll find the tools you need to restore your good health.

The journey starts with understanding just a little bit about how your body works and some of the major issues that have interfered with our health in recent years. Then, in subsequent chapters, you'll find your pathway back to feeling well in both body and mind.

It's important at this point for me to note who this book is for—and who it isn't for. It *is* for those who currently feel depleted and unhealthy, and for whom the system of prescriptions and surgeries and devices has not provided authentic health. This book draws on a belief that all individuals should be equipped with the tools necessary for optimizing their health so they can focus on their life's unique purpose. That's why you'll find here a sensible program for using your body properly, eating real, unprocessed foods in appropriate portions, managing stress, and sleeping in a restorative, healthful way. This isn't a fad diet. This plan is based in evidence and in broad and deep experience on the habits and behaviors that facilitate genuine health.

At the same time, this book is *not* primarily written to doctors or research scientists. I provide here a broad overview of topics that are extraordinarily complex and about which there is always new information. This book is not comprehensive, and it's not meant to be a precise, scientific text.

Nor is this primarily a guide to fast weight loss. There are a million such guides and diets and programs out there. If what you're after is simply shedding pounds and looking better in a swimsuit, then, while this will work, it isn't the right resource for you. If, on the other hand, you want to truly become healthy—and probably also leaner and stronger—then you've come to the right place.

FOR STARTERS, SOMETHING'S WRONG

Between 1960 and 2010, the average American gained approximately thirty pounds. Across our population, we're carrying more adipose tissue—that is, fat tissue—on our bodies than we were two generations ago. That change also has contributed to the diseases that are now at record-setting prevalence, including type 2 diabetes, chronic reflux, irritable bowel, chronic inflammatory pain conditions, and fatigue syndromes, among others.

There isn't a consensus about precisely why we've seen this uptick in obesity and related problems across our population. Some theorize that it is due to technological changes and the way we've become more sedentary. However, evidence has not supported this theory. Our chronic stress levels definitely seem to be impacting our weight. Exactly how, we cannot say for sure. However, as discussed later in this book, I believe we can surmise the reason. One thing that's very clear though, is that our diets have changed, and the change has affected our weight. We'll go into more detail about diet in Chapter Seven, but for now, it's important simply to recognize that the fundamental sources of our nutrition have changed. The quality of the food we eat is different, and how the food is produced is different. How it's preserved is different. How we eat it is different. The proportions of carbohydrates and fats and the amount of sugar in our diet have all fundamentally changed. And there's no doubt that the increase in sugar in our diet—which is a result of the industrialization of food—is a contributor to obesity.

We have been taught to overeat processed foods and to eat them too frequently. We have been influenced into an unnatural pattern of eating. This has caused hormonal changes in our bodies that foster the development of obesity and type 2 diabetes. Our approach to eating is causing these diseases. Do not believe the arguments that obesity is solely the result of overeating and a lack of exercise. Our bodyweight and metabolism are definitely influenced by our calorie intake and our calorie expenditure. But the causes of obesity are genetic and hormonal. Obesity is a multifactorial disease. Our habits influence it, but they are not the primary cause of it. However, the right habits can begin to correct the underlying hormonal issues causing obesity.

There is a massive industry that's supposedly trying to provide us with the "solution" to this problem. You've probably tried a few diets, programs, or supplements to lose weight and improve your health. This is an industry that's making a ton of money by promising that we'll soon look our best, thanks to some new diet or product.

Yet the vast weight-loss and supplement industry is not the answer to your health problems. The truth is that you don't need dietary supplements. If you follow a plan for genuine health—like the one in this book—then you will not need supplements to be healthy or lose weight. And while some of the weight-loss programs may offer some decent information, such as exercise or a healthy nutrition plan, many of them don't. And it's very difficult for consumers to tell the difference.

Still more important, the focus of all these products and programs is almost never on genuine health. The entire industry is centered on looking good by losing weight, very often in an unsustainable manner. A nutrition or exercise program that's about *appearances* instead of health is going to provide the wrong answers because it's asking the wrong questions. Vanity is a shallow motivator, and our looks naturally change over time. The true, underlying motivation has to be your own good health. You don't need devices, gimmicks, or any other product that you can buy at a big-box store. You just need to understand a bit about the fundamental determinants of health, and then you'll need to take action in accordance with that understanding. You don't need weight loss; you need authentic health. Weight loss will follow.

In addition to the diet industry, there's also a whole industry dedicated to selling you pharmaceuticals to manage your poor health. These pharmaceuticals generally aren't aimed at curing the *causes* of your discomfort; instead, they're meant to help you continue to live with that discomfort. A famous example is a heartburn medicine that's advertised in catchy TV commercials with a popular comedian. This comedian tells us that we shouldn't let heartburn come between us and our favorite foods. Often, there's a picture of something like a colossal corndog at the county fair. This pharmaceutical company, of course, is profiting handsomely from that medicine.

But it's deeply troubling that we live in a time when a pharmaceutical company, which is primarily focused on making profit for its shareholders, tells consumers *not* to change potentially harmful habits and instead to buy a product that will help them avoid the consequences of bad food choices. It's especially perverse because those colossal corndogs and other processed foods bring far worse effects than simply heartburn, including arterial disease and cancers.

Can you imagine if a pharmaceutical company ran an ad with a celebrity holding up a pack of cigarettes along with a COPD inhaler, saying that he's not going to let shortness of breath keep him from his favorite cigarette brand? The public would be outraged, and those commercials would be taken off the air.

Well, this is no different. Those unhealthy foods are killing us, and in the same way that tobacco companies are clearly not invested in your health, neither are some of the pharmaceutical companies. Besides encouraging you to eat an unhealthy diet, they're promoting a heartburn medication that also can have serious side effects. When taken over time, that medication will limit your absorption of vitamins and minerals and could then compromise your bone health and lead to osteoporosis. It may also be a contributing factor to dementia and chronic kidney diseases.

Is that how we want to go through life? Do we want to eat foods that have terrible consequences for our bodies and then take prescription drugs that cause still more damage? Or do we desire something better?

In this book, we're equipping you to become your own health advisor.

The story of this book lies in developing habits and behaviors that are consistent with the way your body is truly designed to work. The point isn't weight loss, but if you follow the guidelines of this book, you'll more than likely lose weight. (In fact, recent evidence has suggested that focusing on weight loss alone is not a pathway to regaining health; this has been reported in major publications like *The New York Times*.)

You may look better as a result of the program in this book. But most of all, you will *feel* better—and that's what we're after.

THE CRASH COURSE IN PHYSIOLOGY
THAT EVERYONE SHOULD READ

You're about to learn a few important facts about your body and the ways that our modern eating habits and overall lifestyles have created some significant health problems. Keep in mind that this is only a crash course; it isn't meant to be an exhaustive description of these complicated issues. Instead, you'll find some key information that will help you make healthy choices going forward. It is important to explore what we mean by physiology.

Your body is amazingly complex. Think about this for a moment. All of these dynamic, organic, and infinitely sensitive systems work together to maintain a state of homeostasis, or equilibrium. If everything is functioning well, you experience health. What is health? Well, it can mean many things, but for our purposes, it is you experiencing all of the physical, cognitive, and emotional vitality you have within you. It is you feeling good and pursuing your purposes in life. If your systems are not functioning well, due to many possible reasons, your experience will be less than that of health. You may be actually sick or dealing with diseases, or maybe just lacking the vitality we just mentioned. Your physiology, the functioning of all of your systems, is creating your health.

Your physiology is constantly sending messages to your thinking and feeling centers in your brain. What you are feeling in a given moment is an interpretation of all of the messages being sent to you by your body. How you feel is determined by how you interpret these messages. The messages may be that something is wrong, and you need to feel that. Sometimes the messages are that all is fine but your interpretation is still that something is wrong. Just as your body is sending messages to your brain, your brain is sending messages to your body. If your interpretations are wrong, you can send a message back to the body that something is wrong. That message impacts your physiology. Your physiology impacts your thinking and your thinking impacts your physiology. Both body and mind need to be truly healthy, but they must also be in agreement that you *are* truly healthy. When that is the case, you feel well and are well. This creates well-being.

Your body is constantly taking in information, and your mind continually is interpreting this information. Everything is information. The foods you eat and how often you eat them, whether you are physically active or not, your stress levels, the amount of sleep you get, your environment; all of these are messages to your body. The question is, what messages are your habits sending your body? Are you telling it to be stressed and have its flight-or-fight systems activated? Is your lack of physical activity telling your body that your muscles and bones are not needed? Are the quantities and types of foods you are eating telling your body to store fat or conserve energy? Your body is simply doing what you and your environment are telling it to do. It cannot do anything else.

Now some of these messages are not under your control. However, many, if not most, are absolutely subject to your decision about whether to control them or not. The question is, do you want to control them? In any given moment, your body is giving you the version of yourself that you messaged it to give you. You cannot control all of the variables that affect your being. Your genes are your genes. However, you can influence how those genes express themselves. Your past, and whatever it has done to you, happened, and you have to live with the impact of anything that happened in your past. However, your future is still being written. You have a say in it.

If you want your physiology to support your desires for your future, then you will need to provide the right messages, the right information. If you are careless about those messages, do not be surprised when you experience something other than your best health. At the same time, if you have been taught the wrong messages, how could you possibly experience your best health? Shame and guilt will not help you create the right messages.

Do a short exercise for me. Before reading further, stop and think for a few minutes about the messages your habits are sending your body. Write it down if you can. Really contemplate your desires for your health and what messages your body needs to support those desires. Here is an example of such questions. What message am I giving my body with my current eating habits? Am I telling it that it is worthy of the best nutrition? What nutritional habit could I adopt to send my body a message that I value its function and want it to perform well for me?

◆ Your energy comes from the nutrients you eat

Energy is what fuels our bodies and minds, and we produce it by taking the nutrients from the foods we eat and combining them with the oxygen we breathe and the fluids we drink. In this way, your food becomes the energy that powers you through each and every day.

Our bodies can use any fundamental macronutrient for energy, whether that is an amino acid, a fatty acid, or a simple sugar. The human body's primary energy sources are fatty acids and glucose. Our brains and red blood cells use primarily glucose for energy. Our brains do not use fatty acids for fuel. In the typical American diet, the brain is primarily using glucose from the foods we eat for energy. In fasting states or when following ketogenic diets, the brain will also use ketone bodies for fuel, but it still needs some glucose which can be made from fatty acids and amino acids in a process called gluconeogenesis. While carbohydrates are a source of energy for your body, they are not an essential source. Your body is capable of making its own carbohydrates for fuel.

◆ A healthy body stores energy and then uses that energy later

In normal, healthy circumstances, you consume a meal, and that meal potentially contains complex starches, healthy fats, and protein. Your digestive system then breaks down that meal into amino acids, simple sugars, and fatty acids. But since the meal contained more calories than your body needs as fuel in the precise moment you ate it, your body has to have a way of managing the surplus nutrients.

This is what I am referring to as the "fed" state. In this state, you are diverting energy to digestion and absorption of nutrients. In the fed state, you are also storing nutrients including fatty acids. If you already have enough stored glucose, any excess glucose or fats will be stored as fat in the fed state. The body must have nutrients to function, so you must enter the fed state on a routine basis to be healthy.

Insulin serves many purposes, but one of them is to be the messenger that tells your body what do with all the macronutrients you've just consumed. So insulin tells your body to store excess fatty acids in your cells when you eat. The point of that storage is to save those fatty acids so they will be available later as a source of energy when you are not putting energy into your body through eating.

Insulin also sends signals to other areas, in addition to your fat tissue. It tells cells to take up amino acids and build with them. It sends signals to your muscles and liver to take up glucose and fatty acids and use them for energy or store them as glycogen and fat. In very simple terms, insulin's job is to be released when we eat, tell the food where to go, and then get out of there. That job is very important; without insulin, we die. But you'll see in a second that insulin can play a maladaptive role in our body in response to our modern diet.

When our bodies are in the fed state we use fats and sugars we have just eaten for energy. The surplus amounts of sugars will be stored as glycogen in the liver and muscles and the surplus fats stored as triglycerides in our muscles and adipose (fatty) tissues. In between meals, the body will release stored fuel and use it for the energy necessary to support metabolic functions. It can use both stored fats and stored sugars. It will primarily use the stored sugars from our glycogen. Converting glycogen back to glucose for energy is a quick metabolic process.

The state in between meals when your body is using stored fuels is what I refer to as the "fasting" state. The fasting state is when you have used the available nutrients in your bloodstream, and now your body is utilizing stored nutrients for fuel. The fasting state is a normal state and our bodies are well designed for this. Our fasting states are energy utilizing states. We are using our nutrients to fuel our mind and bodies so we can do whatever needs to be done. This is the state where we should spend most of our time. This is the state where we are generally being productive. The fed state is a time of storage and recovery. The fasting state is a time of action. There are shades of gray with this of course, but as a general principle, it is true.

The body has far more energy stored as fat than it has stored as glycogen. The typical person can fuel their metabolism for 24-36 hours with their glycogen. Vigorous exercise depletes our glycogen more quickly. However, we have enough stored fat, even in lean individuals, to fuel our metabolism for weeks or even months. Severely obese individuals may have enough stored fuel to keep their bodies working for many months.

Your body has everything it needs to manage fasting states without compromising your health. You are supposed to be able to enter into fasting states without psychological stress. They are a normal part of our lives. In fact, in our time, most people never create the need for the body to access it's own fatty acids for fuel. High frequency eating provides a steady stream of calories for energy. With high frequency eating, we stay in a fed state and have no need for our stored fuel. Most people are using glucose from a recent meal and occasionally dipping into their glycogen while they sleep. They are not even coming close to the threshold where their body would need to start using its stored fat as a fuel. You have plenty of energy stored on your body. You just need to approach eating in a manner consistent with how your body is designed to access that energy. It is not that hard to do once you understand how.

I know this chapter may come across as a bit repetitive. Please stay with me through this section of the book. I believe this information is important to understand. Once you know how your body is supposed to work, you will not need a lot more information to be healthy.

Our approach to eating has been so heavily influenced by marketplace dynamics that it is hard to know how to eat. Eating is natural and should not be so confusing. The body is resilient and can pretty much survive in all different types of circumstances. We do not need to be fearful about food. It is only with sustained exposure to harmful stimuli that we lose our ability to stay healthy. Eating in accordance with our design should be intuitive for us.

The thing is, we do have to eat. We do not have to use tobacco or drugs, but we do have to eat. You cannot adopt an abstinence approach to food the way you can with harmful substances. You have to work out what food is for you.

We have been conditioned to eat, eat, and eat some more. Even when we are not hungry, we are told we should eat, that missing a meal is unhealthy. We were taught to eat three meals a day. Then we were taught to add snacks or eat six meals a day. We have been influenced to believe that it is dangerous to go more than a few hours without entering the fed state.

This is simply not true. This approach to eating ignores the necessity of our body entering into fasting states for proper energy utilization.

When our grandparents emphasized our need to eat, they did so from a perspective of having experienced authentic food scarcity. When food is scarce, and the demands of life are intense, if you have the opportunity to eat, then you eat. The threat our grandparents faced was not being able to enter the fed state often enough. That is not the threat we face. The threat we face is not entering into the fasting state often enough.

Our basal metabolism is the sum total of the functions necessary to stay alive each day. We need enough energy to think, to move, to digest, to breathe, to circulate blood, and many other functions. Depending on the messages we send our body in the form of nutrition, movement, stress responses, and sleep, our metabolism can increase or decrease. This is primarily mediated by hormones. However the messages created by our habits strongly influence these hormones. When we have a higher metabolism, we use more calories every day to stay alive. When we have a lower metabolism, we use less calories every day to stay alive. Your body has the ability to use more energy or less energy every day based on the messages it is receiving.

Interestingly enough, it takes a higher metabolic rate to support an obese body. The extra body mass uses more energy. You can have a high metabolic rate and still be obese. In fact, the higher metabolic rate of obese individuals actually increases their appetite. Appetite is strongly influenced by hormones. Obese people upregulate hormones that stimulate appetite. Much of their overeating is based on their hormones, not a deficiency in their self-control. The amount of stored fat a person has is primarily due to genetics and hormones. The genetics and hormones are strongly influenced by what they eat, how much they eat, and how *often* they eat.

Again, in the fed state, we are primarily using what has been eaten and storing the rest. In the fasting state, we are using our stored fuels to support metabolic functions.

One of the major contributors to our obesity problem is we are spending virtually all of our time in the fed state. We eat too much, but we also eat *too often*. Our bodies are designed to do just fine for extended periods of time without food. We cannot survive long without water, but we can survive a very long time without food. For millennia, human beings have been able to fast without compromising their ability to survive. Human beings have always had periods of fasting and feasting. These days, all we do is feast.

We have trained our bodies to stay in a state of perpetual energy storage. Since we can only store a certain amount of fuel as glycogen, you can guess where the rest of it is stored. Yep, it is stored as fat. It does not matter what you have eaten, any excess fuel can be stored as fat. Excess fat becomes fat and excess sugar becomes fat. The major signaling hormone to store food as fat is insulin. When insulin is elevated, your body will continue to store fatty acids in your fat cells rather than releasing them to be used as energy. Persistently elevated insulin levels contribute to weight gain. High frequency eating increases our exposure to insulin.

Your body is supposed to use the nutrients you eat for energy and store the rest, and then use the stored fuel for periods of fasting in between meals. That is how it is designed to work. Insulin is supposed to do its job after we eat and then exit stage left and let some other messengers get to work. That is what is supposed to happen when you eat healthy foods in appropriate portions with appropriate timing of meals.

◆ Our modern diet prevents us from using our stored energy

Over the past decades, our diet has changed to include more processed grains, starches that are less fibrous, a dramatically larger quantity of sugar, and unhealthy industrialized fats. That means the basic nutrients and energy that we put into our bodies has fundamentally changed. Essentially, our foods have become calorie dense and nutrient poor. Instead of putting essential nutrients into our body that give us health and energy, we end up consuming foods that create internal stress and promote nutrient deficiencies. Our food is literally making us sick and actually not providing what our bodies need to function well. This is true for our children as well. Our food is often sending the wrong message to our bodies.

Since we now tend to maintain diets that are heavy in sugar, processed carbohydrates, and industrialized fats, and our portions and snacking have increased, we are consuming excess energy and doing so too often. This creates an energy balance that favors storing energy in the form of fat. The higher concentrations of sugars and processed carbohydrates in our diets cause us to release insulin, and our high frequency eating keeps the insulin high.

Frequent eating of processed carbohydrates and refined sugars causes a *persistently high* level of insulin which favors fat storage. Unfortunately, *persistently high* levels of insulin also influence our neuro-hormonal set point for regulation of our fat storage. Persistently high insulin strongly influences obesity.

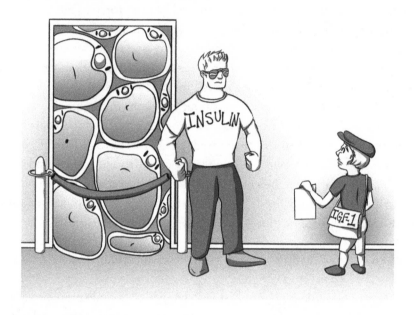

Now, remember that we just covered how our fat cells store energy that should be available for use during periods of fasting. Our adipose tissue is a metabolically active tissue that helps regulate our appetite and our energy balance. Our stored fat is supposed to play an important role in our health. Unfortunately, our modern habits have created a dysfunctional storage system. Now rather than supporting our health and survival, our stored fat is growing on us and creating a diseased state in the body. It is only storing fuel and never releasing it for use.

For adipose tissue to release fatty acids for the production of cellular energy, it has to respond to a complex admixture of messenger hormones. For purposes of simplification, I am describing just one of those, a hormone called "insulin-like growth factor 1," or IGF-1. The actual process is far more complex than I am describing. This IGF-1 is one of the messengers that tells your fatty tissue to release fatty acids into your bloodstream so you can use them as fuel. But as it turns out—thanks to our sugar-heavy diets and the higher insulin levels that results—IGF-1 can't do its job, because all the excess insulin actually interferes with IGF-1's message to your fatty tissue. IGF-1 is trying to tell your body to release those stored fatty acids, but insulin prevents that message from being delivered and instead tells your body to hold onto that fuel.

So picture your fat cell. It's full of fuel. What's more, if you're overweight or obese, that fat cell is holding way too much fuel—which frustrates you. You can't seem to get it to release that fat. Now picture the insulin in your system. It keeps telling that fat cell to hold that fuel. And then picture IGF-1. It's trying to give that fat cell the correct message-to release the stored fat for energy, but insulin will not allow the message to get through. The hormonal messengers that help your body use stored energy cannot get their job done.

◆ Without the ability to use stored energy, we end up eating even more

As if all of that weren't bad enough, the picture gets even worse when you consider the effects of not being able to utilize stored energy properly.

Your adipose tissue is involved in regulating your appetite and your metabolism. As you accumulate excessive fatty tissue, it impacts your ability to manage your hunger. With high levels of insulin, you stay in a fat-storing state. This stored fat is supposed to signal your brain that you are full and keep you from eating. However, the satiety signaling process also ends up disrupted due to multiple factors including resistance to the hormones that signal fullness and activation of your brain's reward system causing you to want to eat more. You still feel hungry even though you have far too much fuel stored on your body. It's a challenging cycle to break. Because you are in a perpetual fat storing state, the systems involved in releasing fatty acids from your fat cells become down-regulated and less active. Your body stops using fats for fuel and uses mostly sugar. Your fat releasing system becomes dormant. Your body is in a state of all storage and no release. This is not good. The only fuel your body can use is sugar. You have lost a key feature of your body's design-metabolic flexibility.

Meanwhile, insulin levels remain high. Over time, your cells stop listening to the insulin. This is called insulin resistance and it is a primary mechanism involved in developing type 2 diabetes. Because insulin is an important messenger for cells to take up glucose and use it for energy, insulin resistance causes your cells to stop taking up the glucose and it remains in the blood stream. Because the glucose is not going where it is needed, your pancreas makes more insulin. The higher levels of insulin basically force the glucose uptake process to occur. Your cells finally take up glucose for use which is good, but your fat cells also continue to store fat. Your rising insulin levels continue to influence weight gain and obesity.

Picture your little brother. He likes to pester you. You learn how to ignore him. What does he do? He doubles his efforts. Little brothers do not give up, they escalate their efforts to get the response they desire. Your insulin is not reduced when your cells do not respond to it. Your insulin is increased. This increases insulin resistance which further increases insulin which increases weight gain. Are you starting to get the idea of what the problem is?

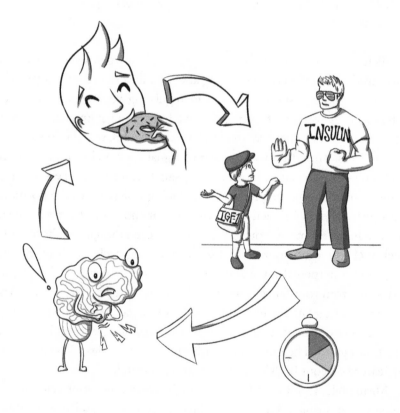

Since most of our modern snacks have sugars and processed carbohydrates, the cycle repeats itself again and again. You eat a sugary snack, insulin swarms in, and it tells your fat cells to store more of that fuel. Your ability to use your stored fuel is compromised. Your appetite is no longer regulated properly. What do you do? You look for a snack to eat.

To make matters still more complicated, many of the snacks we eat today have been specifically engineered to become addictive. Food companies employ scientists to continually invent new products that please our taste buds in such a way that we want to keep on eating them. Those scientists are so good at their jobs that we often develop an emotional attachment to our snacks. Meanwhile, these engineered foods tend to be unhealthy for us in the worst ways: heavy in sugar and full of industrialized fats. There is definite evidence that sugary foods activate the reward system in the brain. This leads to craving for more sugar. We discuss this in more detail in Chapter 5. Truly nutritious foods like fresh vegetables do not activate your reward system. Nutrient dense, fiber-rich foods lower in calories actually increase satiety signaling in your brain causing you to feel satisfied and full. They naturally regulate appetite. They send healthy messages to your body.

So we're not only dealing with a crisis in which our approach to eating has changed our internal hormonal signaling to favor fat storage, but we're also battling the psychological aspects of craving and eating. And that brings us right up to where we are today, with obesity and diabetes at record-setting levels—and only worsening as time ticks on. Even our children are dealing with this problem.

◆ To makes matters worse, visceral fat triggers inflammation

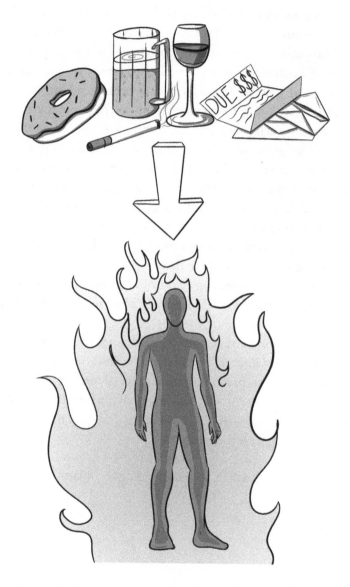

One of your body's natural responses to injury and stress is inflammation. In this process, your body brings various substances to the site of an injury in order to help rebuild tissue or fight infection. That's a normal, healthy occurrence in your body's physiology.

But certain foods and substances, as well as excess bodily fat, can initiate inflammatory responses within your body. Our excessive body fat is pro-inflammatory. Our frequent consumption of sugary and fatty foods increases insulin, which increases accumulation of fat, which increases inflammatory responses in the body. This inflammation contributes to chronic diseases that cause fatigue and pain. This inflammation contributes to cardiovascular diseases, autoimmune diseases, and cancer. It damages our brains and impacts our cognitive functions. Other substances that trigger inflammation include tobacco products, environmental toxins, illicit drugs, and excessive alcohol. Chronic mental and emotional stress can lead to certain hormonal processes that create inflammation. Three of the most inflammatory foods we consume are refined sugars, processed grains, and industrialized vegetable oils. These foods make us sick much like smoking cigarettes. It just happens slowly.

The problem, and the solution, is in our habits. If we continue to overeat processed grains, refined sugars, unnatural oils, artificial dyes, and heavily preserved foods, we'll increase the unhealthy excess fatty tissue that is contributing to inflammation. That means we'll continue to deal with chronic diseases and the uncomfortable symptoms associated with them. In addition, these inflammatory responses make us even more prone to retaining weight and make it difficult for our bodies to function in a healthy, natural way.

THE DIETING CYCLE AND
CONFUSION ABOUT THE THYROID

In recent years the ketogenic, or low-carbohydrate, diet has grown in popularity. A lot of books have been written on the subject, and there is considerable evidence that this type of diet may be a good option for people to improve their weight and their health. It is often referred to as nutritional ketosis.

Essentially we found that by putting chronically obese individuals on a nutrition plan that virtually eliminated all sugars and starches, we would see that, within two to three weeks, sometimes longer, they would go into what's called "ketosis." In a state of ketosis, their bodies were now primarily using fatty acids for fuel. The process of converting from primarily using carbohydrates for fuel to primarily using fatty acids is referred to as fat adaptation. Earlier, we discussed that in our fat storing state, we down regulated the systems that help us use fatty acids for fuel. These systems became dormant. The ketogenic diet, by restricting the consumption of carbohydrates, forces our body to activate the metabolic systems that allow us to efficiently use fatty acids for the energy we need. We can now use our own stored fat as a fuel *if* we actually need to.

Remember, our body will first use what we have eaten for fuel. Also remember that the body can use any macronutrient (amino acids, carbohydrates, fatty acids) to make energy. Therefore, regardless of what we eat, if we consume too many calories we will probably store fat. Also, carbohydrates are not the only initiators of insulin release. Proteins also cause the release of insulin. Artificial sweeteners cause the release of insulin. Many things we consume can initiate the release of insulin. Insulin tells our body to store fat. Even on ketogenic diets, if we eat too much or eat too often, we will still store fat and not lose weight. Eating too frequently causes weight gain regardless of what you are eating. I know I am being repetitive, but it is very important to understand that our bodies are designed for periods of fasting. I will discuss fasting in more detail in our nutrition chapter. For now, just know that no diet that involves eating as much as you want and as often as you want will likely lead to sustained weight loss.

However, the ketogenic diet is good at forcing the process of fat adaptation to occur. In fact, using a ketogenic diet to initiate ketosis before you begin to reduce your frequency of meals is a great way to make longer periods of fasting easier for you to manage. When you are in ketosis, you are using fatty acids to fuel your liver and muscles. Your brain cannot use fatty acids so it will use ketone bodies. Your liver will also use gluconeogenesis to create the additional glucose needed for brain and red blood cell function. Your stored glycogen will be depleted and unavailable for energy. Your stored fats will be available *if* they are needed. In order to lose weight, you will still have to create the right energy balance regardless of whether you are in ketosis or not. There is actually a two step process that has to occur. First you become fat-adapted (able to use fats for energy), and then you become keto-adapted (able to use ketone bodies for energy). You do have to allow your body time to adapt.

Our metabolic rate determines how much energy we use each day. If all things are stable, then our metabolic rate will basically stay stable. Our body seeks homeostasis and will do what is necessary to maintain an overall stable physiology. If our metabolic rate is reduced, we will use less energy. Prolonged calorie restricted diets lower our metabolic rates. If we under-eat for extended periods of time, we send a message to our body to conserve energy. If our body detects that it will only receive 1200 calories a day, it will use only 1200 calories a day or probably less.

Sustained calorie restricted diets are a message of food scarcity. Your body adjusts to this like it would to famine or drought. It senses that in order to survive, it needs to reduce energy expenditure and up-regulate appetite. It will try to keep its remaining fat stores. It will allow muscle wasting as it senses there is no reason to use energy to search for food as none is probably available. It will use as little energy as possible to survive.

At first, with a reduction in calories, insulin levels may lower, and we may start to use our stored fatty acids as a fuel. We may begin to lose weight. However, if we stay in a chronically calorie depleted state, our bodies will go into conservation mode. They will stop using our stored fat as a fuel and simply slow our metabolic rate. This is a survival mechanism. It will happen no matter what we do.

If your body was used to using 2000 calories a day, and it is now only getting 1200 a day, it will reduce its energy expenditure by 800 calories a day or more. This energy will be redirected from your basic physiological processes. Your heart will not beat as hard, your hair and nails will grow more slowly, your body temperature will drop, and many other processes will be impacted. Your neuro hormonal system in your brain will signal your thyroid and other systemic hormonal systems to slow your metabolism. You will feel tired, cold, weak, and potentially depressed. You will think you have low thyroid function. You do not. Your thyroid is doing what your brain is telling it to do (This explanation is oversimplified, but you get the point).

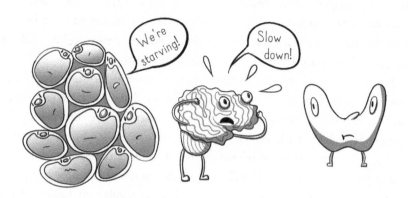

That's why long term calorie restricted diets do not result in *sustained* weight loss. They always fail to provide the results we are seeking. Just as chronically over- eating is unhealthy and causes diseases, chronically un-der-eating is unhealthy and causes diseases. Your energy balance responds to the messages you are providing it.

In addition to this, there is strong evidence that our body fat stores are strongly influenced by genetics. There is a set point our bodies prefer regarding how much stored fuel we maintain. That is why some people can never get the six pack abs they desire. They are not genetically designed to have six pack abs. That is also why many healthy overweight people may not need to lose weight. If they eat healthy foods in appropriate portions, if they exercise, if they get plenty of sleep and manage stress well, and if their health metrics look good, they do not need to lose weight. Their extra body fat is being determined by their genetics. We can influence how our DNA expresses itself, but we cannot change our DNA. Many people the medical system classifies as obese, and then subsequently targets for interventions, are not over-eating or being too sedentary. It is just the way their bodies are designed. It can do more harm than good to tell them they have a weight problem.

Allow me a brief editorial aside. In my medical practice, we have been trying for years to help our patients improve their lifestyle and lose weight to reverse chronic diseases like diabetes. Most health insurance companies would not cover weight loss programs as they were considered cosmetic. Now, the health insurance companies are beginning to recognize that obesity is often a medical disease that needs to be addressed. Of course, their primary concern is the fiscal risk to them if this problem continues to worsen. They are concerned about their pocketbooks, not the health of their members.

If they were concerned about the health of their members, they would provide access to our comprehensive lifestyle approach to treating diseases. Instead, they now want to micromanage how we address obesity with our patients. They want us to report to them the BMI, Body Mass Index, on every patient we see. In addition to that, if the BMI is abnormally high or low, we are supposed to document that we counseled the patient about this. If we do not, it is a negative mark against our quality scores.

Think about this. Your insurance company will not pay for you to address your obesity, but they want your weight reported to them at every visit. They do not care if talking to you about your weight may be more harmful than helpful. They do not care that you are actually having a medical visit for severe depression and talking about your weight will actually make it worse. They do not care that you are being seen for a high fever. They want to make sure you know you are obese and that your doctor told you. "Hi Mrs. Smith. I know you are experiencing lower gastrointestinal bleeding. However, I would like to take a moment and counsel you about your weight."

This is perverse. The same institutions who were supposed to manage our healthcare dollars and look out for our health refused to acknowledge the developing obesity problem in our population. These institutions now want to micromanage a problem they failed to take seriously in the past. The risk managers at your insurance company think they know the best way to manage your obesity problem. They do not believe you will change, and they do not believe your doctor can be trusted to look out for your best interests. That is why you have to become your own health advocate.

THE DIETING CYCLE AND MAINTAINING WEIGHT LOSS

Every person has a genetic set point for weight. Your body will more or less hover around this weight. However, that set point can change over time. We do not yet fully understand how this occurs, but the longer you are overweight or obese, the more likely you create a new set point for your weight. Once the set point is changed upward, it is hard to lower your weight from that point. It can be done, but it is hard. Your body is designed to stay close to the programmed set point for body composition. This is a result of internal hormonal signaling. Your body fat is regulated by hormones. These hormones are influenced by your habits.

This is part of the reason that diets eventually fail. Our bodies seek to regain the weight that has been lost. It will do this even if we continue many of the healthy lifestyle changes we have made. Once you lose a certain amount of body fat, your metabolic rate will drop and your hunger will increase. You regain your weight. This is the point where we often blame the patient for not following the program. Much of the time, that is not true. The patient follows the program, but the program does not work. Rather than examine whether our program actually works, we blame the patient. It is easier than admitting our approach to weight loss may be ineffective.

This may make it seem as though it is not even worth trying to lose weight. What is the point if we are just going to regain the weight we lost and perhaps even gain more than we lost?

Actually, there are approaches to nutrition that have evidence they will result in sustained weight loss without having to chronically under-eat. These approaches to eating address the underlying hormonal problems that are causing weight gain and obesity. They address the root causes of the problem, and therefore, are effective at initiating and *sustaining* weight loss. This is good news. We will discuss these approaches in more detail in our nutrition chapter. For now, just know that balancing fed and fasting states is an important part of sustaining weight loss.

It does appear that the set point for weight may be strongly influenced by insulin levels. When we help people with weight loss, they will go through plateaus where their weight loss stalls. If we can help them manage the plateau without regaining their weight, after enough time, their brain accepts the new set point for weight and will allow them to start losing more weight. The more we are able to lower insulin and insulin resistance, the easier it is to maintain steady weight loss.

Ketogenic and low carbohydrate diets help lower insulin levels. These diets help people maintain weight loss. Fasting lowers insulin levels. Fasting helps people maintain weight loss. Properly designed and monitored ketogenic or lower carbohydrate diets combined with intermittent fasting protocols are perhaps the best method of initiating and sustaining weight loss. Once the desired weight has been obtained, and the brain has accepted this new set point, people can experiment with different nutritional approaches to determine what works best for them.

I encourage people to eat the broadest diet they are able that still maintains healthy body weight and helps them feel their best. For some, this is low carbohydrate. For others, it may have a higher percentage of carbohydrates. However, all diets that help maintain weight and overall health involve minimizing or eliminating processed carbohydrates, added sugars, and industrialized vegetable oils. Processed carbohydrates and refined sugars are prompt and potent stimulators of insulin release. As we have discussed, persistently high levels of insulin leads to weight gain.

I work with many patients on the ketogenic diet, but it has become clear that it may not be a comprehensive and sustainable health and weight-loss solution for everyone. However, to initiate weight loss, and as a way of reversing diabetes, it is very effective. Emerging evidence is highly supportive of using low-carbohydrate, ketogenic nutrition plans to reverse diabetes altogether.

I want to be clear that just following a low carbohydrate diet is not necessarily following a ketogenic diet. A ketogenic diet is more complex than just getting rid of carbohydrates and sugars. It is beyond the scope of this book to fully describe the ketogenic diet. However, there are many excellent books that can provide you all of the details of the ketogenic diet. I have provided a summary approach to adopting a ketogenic diet at www. healthshepherds.com.

Each nutritional plan must be individualized, and we have to limit the amount of time that people remain on a very low-calorie diet. Low carbohydrates and low calories will eventually lead to a significant slowing of the metabolic rate—the speed at which we burn calories. We have learned much about obesity and metabolism during the past few years that has helped us improve our approach to using this type of nutrition plan.

Historically, we would place people on a low-carb, low-calorie diet. This would often work and they would lose weight quickly. They would feel so good that they would follow this diet for more than the three months our program called for. Typically, we would want our patients to moderate their diet after about nine weeks and then vary their daily calorie intake rather than maintaining a sustained low calorie diet. Our patients would lose a good bit of weight, but around month six, they would start gaining it back. The only way they could prevent the weight gain was to stay on a lower-calorie, lower-carbohydrate diet. They reported feeling hungry and tired. If they resumed normal eating, they would regain weight rapidly.

This same issue occurred with any type of sustained calorie restriction, whether it was low-carb or low-fat. All diet and exercise plans followed faithfully would result in weight loss. Unfortunately, all of them also resulted in a slowed metabolic rate. This eventually resulted in weight gain back to their body's set point, perhaps even higher.

Something was wrong with our approach. Why would a healthy, forty-something person who is physically active be able to consume only 1,400 calories a day and very minimal carbohydrates in order to maintain his or her weight loss—and at the same time struggle with chronic hunger and fatigue?

We were working off of the wrong theory of weight gain and obesity. We assumed, like everyone else, is was about calories in versus calories out. Calories in and calories out was not the root cause of the problem. The root cause was the changing internal hormonal environment of the body. Our approach, and virtually all others, were excellent to help people lose weight. The problem was not losing weight, it was keeping it off once it was lost. Our solutions needed to address the root cause of the problem.

That's why people found themselves losing weight, gaining weight, losing weight, gaining weight, over and over again. Unfortunately, this ineffective approach to sustained weight loss caused further metabolic derangement to our bodies and also caused a considerable amount of blaming ourselves for our inability to maintain a healthy weight. We did not understand that our own body was working against us because it was getting the wrong messages.

Starting in the 1950's and escalating in the 1970's, our approach to eating became unnatural. We were encouraged to eat a high carbohydrate diet with no regard for the sources of those carbohydrates. They could be from refined sugars, processed grains, corn, or any other starch. We were encouraged to stop eating fats and start eating carbs. In order to improve the affordability of this, our government heavily subsidized the production of wheat and corn. Processed foods were cheap, convenient, tasty, and presumably good for us. Unfortunately, processed carbohydrates and refined sugars were unnatural. All of the fiber, protein, and fat associated with them was removed. All that was left was a highly absorbable starch that caused a prompt increase in blood glucose, and therefore, insulin. We also replaced healthy natural fats with unhealthy highly processed fats that were pro-inflammatory. We were also encouraged to eat more frequently. We were told to have snacks in between meals and always eat breakfast.

These two eating behaviors-consumption of processed foods and high frequency eating-caused a hormonal response that favors weight gain and obesity. These two behaviors were inconsistent with our approach to eating for almost all of recorded human history. Look at any graph that shows the velocity with which our population has become obese over time. It will tell you the truth about this. Our obesity problem started when we started eating a lot of carbs, sugars, and vegetable oils, and eating them frequently. This is not just based on population health evidence, this is common sense.

That is why we witnessed so much successful weight loss using lower carbohydrate approaches. As we lowered carbohydrates, we were lowering insulin and hastening fat adaptation. However, even those strictly adhering to lower carbohydrate diets often experienced difficulty maintaining weight loss. Eventually they struggled as well. Many of my patients who followed a long term low carbohydrate diet eventually regained their weight.

We described above some of the reasons for this. We now have a better understanding about the genetic influencers of obesity. We understand how the body reacts to weight loss and seeks to regain the weight. We understand how long term calorie restriction leads to a slowing of the metabolic rate and an increase in hunger. However, there are other reasons why these diets do not work for everyone.

One of those is that carbohydrates are not the only initiators of insulin release. Proteins increase insulin. Artificial sweeteners increase insulin. Even fats cause a small increase in insulin. Eliminating carbohydrates alone as a primary approach to sustained weight loss did not fully address the underlying hormonal issues causing our weight problems.

Also, for many people, a low carbohydrate diet is just not sustainable. There are a couple reasons for this. One reason is very intuitive: any diet that cuts out an entire food group, or food groups, is going to be challenging over the long term. There are social pressures that make it difficult to cut out sugar and starch in perpetuity. On top of that, it's just plain hard to eliminate a group of foods that you enjoy.

Our bodies do not have to use carbohydrates for fuel. We can survive just fine without them. However, we live in a time where carbohydrates are cheap and available. Whether that is how it should be or not is irrelevant. It is our reality. Most people are going to consume some carbohydrates as part of their diet. If we can get them to choose fibrous non-processed carbohydrates and avoid added sugars, then we can still help them reverse their obesity and chronic diseases. Ketogenic diets are a fast track to this result. But we *can* get there following a more balanced approach if that is what has to be done.

The only diet that is good for you is one that is sustainable for you. However, if the only diet sustainable for you includes high frequency consumption of processed carbs and sugars, then you will not correct the messages you are sending your body. Your sustainable diet still has to be a healthy one. But it does not have to be a low carbohydrate diet. You can still lower insulin levels while eating a diet containing all of the macronutrients. Especially if you are willing to consider fasting.

There is no doubt that our strong cravings for carbohydrates and sugars and our inability to control our consumption of them is maladaptive in our current food abundance paradigm. Why is it so hard to resist the consumption of foods that are causing weight gain and disease? Most non-smokers do not have cravings for cigarettes because they know how bad they are for them. Why are we so overwhelmed by our desires to eat foods that are toxic for our health? The regulation of our hunger and our cravings is a major issue impacting our energy balance. We will cover this in more detail throughout the book. For now, know that often our hunger is not actually associated with a need for food. It is a conditioned response in our brain from our overeating and eating too often. It is also strongly influenced by internal signals that are not under our conscious control.

Hunger has both psychological and hormonal roots. You have to address both your psychological cravings and your hormonal signaling to gain control over hunger. Snacking increases hunger, it does not satisfy it. Frequent meals and snacking do not increase our metabolism or reduce our hunger. Most of our snacking involves processed foods and sugars. This triggers increased insulin which increases fat storage. These unhealthy snacks also trigger hunger. They make us want to eat more.

There is a hormone called leptin which is produced by fat cells that's supposed to help with satiety. There are many satiety hormones, but leptin is a major one. As fatty tissue increases, leptin increases, which is supposed to signal us to eat less. Obese people have very high levels of leptin, yet they continue to feel hungry. It appears that, as our fatty tissue increases, we become resistant to the message of leptin. Therefore our appetite becomes improperly regulated.

We have to deal with our hunger. If we are not willing to go through the discomfort of getting control of our hunger, we will not be able to maintain a healthy weight. When we are in ketosis, we tend to feel much less hungry. Learning how to fast helps us gain mastery over the sensation of hunger. Fasting is a fast track to mastering hunger. It is like pulling the bandage off quickly. It is uncomfortable, but it gets the job done.

Fasting also does not slow our metabolic rate the way long term calorie restriction does. Actually, when we fast, a number of positive hormonal and metabolic processes occur. We lower insulin. We increase growth hormone. We increase the activity of our sympathetic nervous system which increases our metabolic rate and eventually reduces our hunger. If we are not on blood sugar lowering medications, we do not develop low blood sugar. Fasting does not cause hypoglycemia (for those who do not have medical hypoglycemia). Most people falsely believe that is does. It does not. Our blood sugar is maintained through releasing our glycogen stores and eventually through gluconeogenesis. Once we have depleted our glycogen, we begin to up regulate the process of using our stored fat as a fuel. We hasten fat adaptation by fasting. We become capable of using our stored fats as a fuel.

Fasting is quite good for us and it is good for our metabolism. When done properly, it is safe for most people. There are some who should not fast, but most can. Our bodies are designed to maintain our strength and energy while enduring periods of low food intake. This makes sense. A brief period of food deprivation should increase our energy so we can go hunt and gather. It is only over the last decades that we have been consistently messaged that fasting is dangerous or unhealthy. This is simply not true. There is no evidence that fasting is unsafe. The dietary recommendations we have been taught over the past decades have been heavily influenced by food manufacturers. Food manufacturers make money selling us food. Food manufacturers do not make money when we fast. In fact, no one makes money when we fast. Food manufacturers want us to eat a lot of food and to eat often. There is not a shred of evidence to support that we need to eat snacks to be healthy.

Fasting can help us lose weight, reverse diseases like obesity and diabetes, and improve our metabolic functions. Fasting can help lower insulin levels for those who want to eat diets with higher percentages of carbohydrates. Fasting is a healthy habit. Almost everyone should learn to fast. For millennia, fasting was an essential survival skill for human beings to endure periods of low food availability. Now, we have found out that fasting is an essential skill to survive a time in which food is far too plentiful. I have created a mini book that provides more details about how to adopt a fasting practice that can be found at www.healthshepherds.com.

Long term calorie restricted diets lead to lower metabolic rates, regaining of weight, and fatigue. The message of long term calorie restriction to your body is to go into an energy conservation state. The message of fasting is to go into an energy utilizing state. It is important to understand this distinction which is why I am spending so much time on this. In case you are getting nervous about what I mean by fasting, do not be alarmed, we will explain how simple it can be in Chapter 7.

Ultimately, long term weight loss occurs in two phases. The initial phase is facilitated by simply following a program that allows for your body to use your stored fat for fuel. There are many programs that can help with this. However, most of these will not provide what is necessary for long term weight loss. For long term weight loss, we have to reset the set point in your brain for your body fat regulation. This requires addressing the root causes of obesity, the hormonal causes. This requires addressing all of the contributors to obesity.

Unfortunately, the longer we are obese, the harder it is to change our body composition. This is especially important to keep in mind when considering the problem of childhood obesity. Obese children are more likely to be obese adults. They will be more likely to develop the chronic diseases that accompany obesity. The fact that our children are being diagnosed with these diseases should be causing us to closely examine our approach to nutrition. We should not send our children into adulthood already burdened by metabolic diseases. Our approach to eating is giving our kids diseases that they will deal with for the rest of their lives. This is serious. Our children started becoming obese over the past few decades. We must examine what changed in our approach to feeding our children over that time.

Consider the concept of energy balance. This is the equation that determines what your body is doing with its energy. The way you were probably taught to think about this was **Calories In – Calories Out = Energy Balance.** If you consume more energy than you use, you gain weight, and if you consume less energy than you use, you lose weight. It's a pretty simple formula that is not at all an accurate explanation of how our body manages energy. That kind of simplicity may be reasonably accurate for machines, but for infinitely complex human beings, not so much. Your energy balance is subject to the interplay of many complex influencers. Certainly energy in versus energy out is a major influencer, but consider this list of additional influencers: genetics, environment, psychological factors, cultural and sociological phenomena, sleep, stress, hormones, neurotransmitters, enzymes, and many others. You get the idea. Your energy balance is complex.

If you have a problem with your energy balance, and you do not have a disease that directly impacts your energy balance, then it is likely the result of the messages you are sending to your physiology. The message of a sedentary lifestyle is to slow the metabolism. The message of overeating and frequent snacking is to store excess energy. The message of excessive stress is to increase cortisol and ultimately to increase insulin and inflammation. The message of processed foods, refined sugars, and artificial ingredients is to increase inflammatory responses in the body. The message of excessive visceral fat results in insulin resistance, inflammation, dysregulation of appetite, and derangement of normal metabolism.

This is why the re-creation of a normal metabolism and healthy energy balance requires a holistic solution. We must correct all of the messages, not just one or two of them. If you were to pick the two messages that are probably most influential for your energy balance, it would be your nutrition and your stress responses. Approaching nutrition in accordance with your bodies design is an essential habit of health. This must be done. There are many ways to provide the right nutritional message to your body, but it must be done.

Chronic unmitigated stress leads to *persistently high* levels of cortisol. Cortisol increases blood sugar which increases insulin. Chronic stress leads to weight gain. Even with the right nutritional approach, a chronically stressed person will still struggle with weight gain. Chronic psychological stress is a negative message to your physiology. Chronic stress also depletes your willpower which impacts your habits. Chronic stress is highly subversive to your health. That is why this book teaches you how to master stress before we move into our nutritional chapter.

WE KNOW WHAT IT TAKES
TO KEEP A BODY HEALTHY

So what *is* the answer to our widespread ill health?

The real answer doesn't involve buying brand-new "health" products or supplements, and it doesn't involve crash diets or eliminating a whole food group—except the group that contains highly processed, low-quality foods.

The answer was right in front of us all along. The answer has everything to do with allowing our bodies to operate in accordance with their design—which, by and large, is the way they *were* operating, until just a few decades ago.

We're going to recreate the situation in which your body has the nutrients needed to function properly. We're going to allow your body to become metabolically flexible and use energy properly. While challenging, we hope to recreate your ability to manage your hunger. As you begin to use your stored fat as a fuel, your excess adipose tissue will be reduced and therefore the inflammation in your body will be reduced. Chronic diseases such as type 2 diabetes will be better controlled or altogether reversed. As you become healthier, you will have more energy and feel good. You will regain your health.

In order to do that, you'll need to eat healthy and nutritious foods in appropriate portions. You'll need to maintain some physical activity, and you'll need to get restorative sleep. And to do *those* things, you'll need to change what are likely deeply ingrained habits—which will require paying some attention to your thinking and mindset.

It's important to note that you'll need to do *all* of these things, not just a few of them, in order to get your body truly back to a healthy rhythm. Nutrition alone isn't going to solve your problem; you're going to need the right nutrition in tandem with the right physical use of your body as well as effective stress management. It is okay to make small changes over time, but all areas have to be addressed. You'll understand precisely why you need all of these elements, as opposed to just one or two of them, as you read on.

Will this be worth it? Absolutely. As you create the habits that send the messages of health and vitality to your physiology, you will begin to experience energy and well-being. You will be able to maintain a healthy body weight (in accordance with your genetics). You will have mental, emotional, and physical energy. You will reduce the impact of chronic diseases on your health. You will reduce or eliminate the need for medicines. You will live longer and with a higher quality of life. You will be more productive in your personal and professional life. You will properly value health as one of the most important attributes you possess. You will not give it away to unfulfilling and energy draining habits. This journey is absolutely worth it. You just have to have an accurate map of how to get where you want to go. This book is that map.

If all of this sounds complicated, or if you already have a lot of questions about exactly how you're going to do all these things, don't worry. You'll find everything you need to know in the pages ahead.

ADDITIONAL RESOURCES

- *The Obesity Code,* by Jason Fung M.D.
- *The Hungry Brain: Outsmarting the Instincts That Make Us Overeat,* by Dr. Stephen Guyenet and Aaron Abano
- Our resources at www.healthshepherds.com

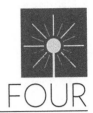

FOUR

To Change Your Health, First Change Your Thinking

This chapter teaches you how to cultivate the mindset that will allow you to apply the rest of the material in this book. You'll learn how to condition your brain to think in a way that supports your best health. You will use the power of your mind to master your habits and optimize your health. You can take control of your thoughts.

IN THIS CHAPTER you'll find the philosophy that underlies everything else in this book. Maybe you're feeling tempted to go straight to Chapter Seven, because you want nutrition tips for losing weight—but this book doesn't work that way. Instead, it's about identifying and influencing the deepest determinants of your health, and your thinking may be the most important determinant of all. If you decide to skip this chapter in favor of other topics, you'll be missing a key ingredient.

Our thought life has amazing power. Our ability to think creatively, intuitively, rationally, and in a manner consistent with our overall well-being differentiates us from all other creatures. Our minds are an amazing gift that are supposed to help us maximize our health so we can serve our purpose. We have the ability to envision the destiny we desire for ourselves and our families. We then have the ability to determine what the necessary steps are to make that destiny our reality. Our minds can then orchestrate our habits and behaviors to see to it that we arrive at that destiny. This is an amazing power and we should put it to good use.

The only way your mind can do this for you is if you take ownership of your thought life. Your mind will always be thinking about something. You can see to it that your mind focuses on your highest desires. I hope your health is one of those desires. If you give up your right to manage your own thought life, your destiny will be determined by others and your behaviors determined by hormones and neurochemicals that you cannot consciously control. If you use your mind rightly, your hormones and neurochemicals will provide your body and mind the messages consistent with your desires. You will choose what you truly desire. You will choose health.

Step number one on your path to good health is simply to become aware. Awareness, intentionality, and mindfulness are all buzzwords today—in large part because we have become so *un*aware and *un*intentional. Our modern-day habits tend to be determined not by our conscious and purposeful choices, but instead by savvy companies with a product to sell, whether that product is a sugary snack, a bacon cheeseburger, a sensational news channel, a new device, or even a fad diet. Our habits are now so strongly influenced by these forces that we're often entirely tuned out of what we're choosing and doing.

So your first step is to begin to develop awareness of what you're choosing and doing. The logic behind this is pretty simple. If there's something about your life that you want to change—as there surely is, or you wouldn't be reading this book—then solving the problem will take a bit of understanding about what the problem is in the first place.

At our core, we human beings are a bundle of habits. At any given moment on any given day, we're all doing what our habits tell us to do. The way your body is physically engaged at this moment is a neurologically based motor habit that you've developed over time—meaning your brain has gotten used to sending certain signals to your body. That's why it's essential for you to become aware. Without awareness, you'll continue to go in whatever direction your habits take you.

Nor is this wisdom just for those who are dealing with acute health problems. Awareness of habit—and how to form new ones in an intentional way—is something that underlies the achievement of many highly successful people.

What's more, in addition to having spent years reading the medical and psychological literature to understand this subject, I personally use this wisdom in my own life every day. I am continually trying to pause and become aware of what I'm doing and why. That's hugely important for me to be an effective and happy father, husband, and doctor supervising a medical team. My guess is that it will soon be hugely important for you, too.

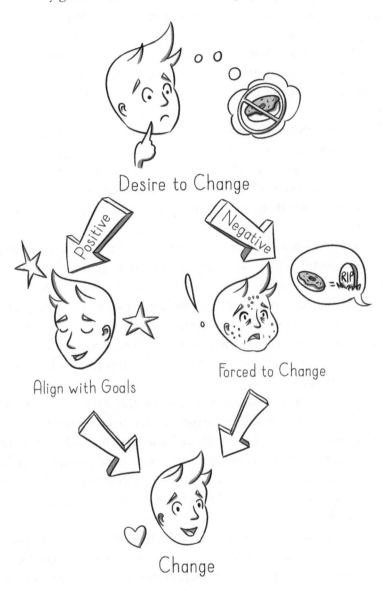

DESIRE AND THE POWER TO CHANGE

You have big-picture desires. If you're like most people, you desire meaningful relationships, peace and contentment, and physical health and vitality. You're probably very clear about the fact that you desire those things. At the same time, you have much smaller, day-to-day desires: you might want a cold beverage right now, or you want to be distracted from a stressor in your life. Sometimes, those smaller desires move us further from, rather than closer to, our larger desires. Does that mean that you want the smaller desires more than the larger ones? Maybe, but not necessarily.

You're not always *choosing* those smaller desires in a conscious way. Sometimes your choices are the result of conditioned responses that are programmed in your brain. Here you start to see why awareness is so essential—because you won't be able to reverse conditioned responses without becoming aware that they're taking place. That's why awareness is the first step.

As you develop awareness, you start to move into a place where you can clearly identify what's happening. You become aware of the fact that you're making the choices you're making. You might also become aware that certain choices run counter to your larger goal of becoming healthy, and yet you're still choosing them. Retraining your brain will take time.

But as you become aware of what's happening, you now have the opportunity to ask yourself, "Why am I choosing this when I know it isn't what I want for myself?"

I've had countless patients who've told me that they really, truly desire good health. So I give them the instructions for how to improve their nutrition and how to become physically active in ways that will provide them health and energy. Then, six months later, those same patients come back to see me—and they haven't changed a thing. Do they really desire good health? Or do they desire something else even more? Once again, awareness is essential.

If you don't truly want authentic health more than you want some of your current day-to-day comforts, then there's nothing and no one who can give your health to you. No one can devise a medication, a supplement, or a product that will give you real health. Some people and companies will tell you they can; they'll tell you that all you have to do is pay the cash price.

But no one has the answer.

The truth is that it's in you. Your doctor can't want it for you. Your spouse can't want it for you. Your kids can't want it for you. Your parents can't want it for you. Your employer can't want it for you. You have to want it for yourself.

So unless you truly desire health, this book will not help you, because you'll have to change some of your habits, and at times, change is difficult. You're going to have to be willing to endure some discomfort. Some things might be easy, and all of it will get easier as you progress, but some of it will be challenging. Some of it may be *very* challenging.

What I can promise you, though, is that you'll be glad for every ounce of effort you put into it. Think about an athlete preparing for a big competition. What do they do? They prepare, they train, and they change their habits. And when they reach their goal, they say it was all worth it. Your health is just like that: You want it, you desire it, and when you've achieved it, you'll say without any doubt that it was worth every bit of effort.

This book helps get you there by providing all the information you need to convert existing habits into healthy ones, from nutrition to physical activity to restorative sleep to stress management. But you'll have to bring a key ingredient. Your job is to *desire* it. You have to want health to be your habit.

CHANGE MUST BE NECESSARY

To achieve the health you're looking for, you'll require two things: necessity and competency. All change happens out of necessity; without necessity, no change occurs.

Necessity can come from positive or negative motivators. A positive motivator might be a person who's so driven by her purpose and goals that she absolutely must have all her energy and health in order to accomplish what she's set out to do. She's not willing to give up her health to bad habits; she'll find health because of that powerful positive motivator.

Meanwhile, a negative motivator might be that a person's current state of being has become intolerable. Maybe it's come to the point where he's so sick all the time—drained of his energy, drained of mental, physical, and emotional health—that he feels he has no choice but to change. At that point, he'll find a way to change.

In addition to necessity, you'll also need competency in order to change. A person with the most profound desire to become healthy still needs to have the ability and crucial information about how to change his habits and behaviors; he has to have the *competency* to become healthy. That can be very difficult in our modern world. If we waited for our food companies to give us the information and competency for making nutritious choices, we would *never* achieve health. Without knowledge of what constitutes healthy choices, you can't get where you want to go. So you need that competency.

In fact, that's why I wanted to write this book. My staff and I realized that we needed a way of offering comprehensive information to our patients so they could acquire the competency to become truly healthy.

NEUROPLASTICITY—AND THE POWER YOU DIDN'T KNOW YOU HAD

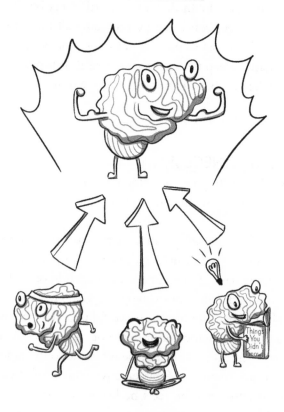

In medical school, I learned that the human brain grows and changes up until a certain point and then, after that, it's basically fixed, with little potential for growth or to repair from damage caused by injury. But it turns out that much of what I learned during medical school about the brain's potential for growth was incorrect.

In actuality, the brain is very plastic. Your brain can adapt, learn, change, and grow throughout your whole life, as recent advances in technologies, such as functional brain imaging, have shown. Your brain, in other words, is extraordinarily powerful. There's really no skill and no competency that it can't help you develop, as long as you have the desire to do it!

Christopher Reeve is a compelling example of this. He was told that his quadriplegia was permanent and that there was no chance he would be able to move his extremities by means of his own efforts ever again. Then he proved doctors and scientists wrong. Before his death, he had developed the ability to initiate movement in his fingers and hips. He proved that, even after a permanent severing of the connections of the body to the brain, the brain is powerful enough to redevelop and initiate those controls.

That's nothing short of astonishing—and it is great news for you, because you, too, have an incredibly powerful brain. It is entirely capable of learning new habits and equipping you with the ability to reach your goals and serve your life's purpose.

Neuroscience has established at least three primary ways to stimulate and grow new neural networks and, thereby, to develop new ways of thinking. In other words, there are three key types of activities that can enhance your neuroplasticity and build your brain:

- **Sustained aerobic activity.** For the purpose of strengthening your brain, aerobic activity ideally should be sustained for forty-five minutes, daily if possible, while disconnected from headphones or other technology so that you can fully engage in what you're doing. Yet if all you can manage to do is fifteen minutes, that will still help—and, if necessary, you can combine it with the second activity...

- **Exercises to practice mental focus and meditation.** These are simple, brief exercises that strengthen and enhance your ability to focus and stimulate the areas of your brain that regulate your

emotions and awareness. (Details at the end of this chapter.)
- **Novel learning experiences.** This is just what it sounds like: learning something new. Whether it's a new language or a new card game, novel learning experiences help to grow your brain.

Currently, your thinking and behaviors are based on your existing wiring, much of which was programmed when you were young. Your way of managing stress and conflict, of being positive or negative in the face of challenges, of being judgmental or nonjudgmental of yourself and others, all has a lot to do with how you're wired. In the short term, that makes us very predictable. Those closest to you can probably guess how you'll respond in a given situation. But in the medium and long term, you can change your wiring.

This is as profound as what's in your DNA—or, more specifically, how your DNA expresses itself. While you can't change your genetic code, the *expression* of that code actually changes continuously in response to your environment, how you think, how you move, what you eat, and what is influencing your emotions. Research in the groundbreaking field of *epigenetics* shows that the expression of certain genes is continuously turned on or off in response to our behavior or environmental factors, in ways that affect our mood, metabolism, weight gain, insulin response, and just about everything else.

When it comes to your mood, let's say that your genetic disposition is about eighty percent toward calmness and composure and twenty percent toward anxiety. Well, if you grow up in a household where everyone is anxious, that minority portion of your genetic code is going to express itself. But if you move yourself toward a peaceful environment, surrounded by peaceful people, and work on meditation, you can change your genetic expression to a calm demeanor. You can choose your destiny; you're not limited by your DNA. You can determine what version of yourself wakes up tomorrow.

In addition to the expression of certain genes over others, some of your existing habits may also have to do with what's called *implicit memory*. As its name implies, we're not consciously aware of our implicit memories. Consider, for instance, a person who grew up with an alcoholic father who tended to get very angry when he was drunk. This person learned at a young age that the best thing to do when he saw signs of anger—a look in his father's face, a certain tone, an abruptness of demeanor—was simply to get away and escape.

As this person grows older, he isn't aware of this ingrained behavior. But he carries with him a memory tied to anger and a wired response that tells him to escape when someone gets angry. He then carries that implicit memory all the way into adulthood. Whenever anyone gets angry—including his spouse—he flees. He doesn't think about why he does it; he just does it. But it's possible for him, together with his spouse and probably a behavioral therapist, to discover the root of that behavior and condition a new response.

That might seem like an extreme example, but it's very much related to your own behaviors and habits. Consider that your behaviors are your behaviors precisely because they feel good in some detectable way to your brain. This is called the "habit loop." It's a three-step loop that develops in the brain in which we (1) encounter a cue or trigger, (2) respond with a particular behavior, and (3) feel a sense of reward from that behavior. In the case of the child fleeing his father, the behavior felt good in the sense that he avoided pain. The reward becomes attached to the behavior, and we become conditioned to respond in that particular way when we encounter the cue.

It can be very difficult to pin down the original cues that led us to form the habits that we have. But even if you can't decipher their origins, it's important to become aware of what are now your habits—with regards to what you eat and drink, how you hold your body all day, how you manage stress, how you spend any spare time, and what you reach for when you're feeling down.

You can also use this information about conditioned behaviors and habits in order to improve your emotional intelligence. When you're tuning in to your actions and feelings, you have an opportunity to start to recognize and understand your emotions. That's the way to develop impulse control and to be able to avoid responding to some situations in an automatic way.

More broadly, you have an astounding potential for change and growth. You have the ability to assess your current habits and automated responses and then to decide whether they're helping or hurting you. If they're hurting you, you can dig deeper. Where did these habits come from? How would you like to change them?

Then you can actually change your brain, and from there you'll change your habits. Yes, it will take effort. It will require awareness, desire, and a willingness to engage in a process that will consume some of your energy and time. But it's well worth it to free yourself from habits that were conditioned into you long ago. You aren't beholden to those old habits; you can *choose* to *choose* your behavior—and when you can do that, you'll be able to choose the life that you'll lead.

THE TRANSFORMATIVE POWER OF PERSPECTIVE

Different perspectives lead to different destinies. If your perspective is negative, then your destiny will be negative. If your perspective is positive, then your destiny will be, too. That might sound like a cliché, and yet by definition, it's true. You're the one judging whether your life is good or bad; a positive outlook will allow you to see your life from a positive standpoint.

It turns out that a significant percentage of our unhealthy behaviors arise from our inability to handle negative or uncomfortable feelings. Psychologists often refer to this as "taking the low road" as we end up lost in our lower mind. I like to reference thoughts and behaviors as either coming from our higher mind or our lower mind. This is a major simplification but it works for most of my patients.

Our higher mind is our most advanced mind. It differentiates us as human beings and allows us to manage our emotions and thoughts. It allows us to become our best selves. It is a powerful processing center in our brain and must be intentionally exercised. It also requires adequate and high quality nutrients to function well. Trust me, you want to activate and strengthen your higher mind. This takes intentional effort. Otherwise, your reactive and reward seeking lower mind will be calling the shots.

Taking the low road typically means feeling shame, guilt, jealousy, self-pity, victimhood, and perhaps, contempt for others. This pattern develops because we desperately want to escape from uncomfortable feelings or emotions—and that desire for escape sends us into habits that might include eating something, drinking something, watching something, or even coming up with a fantasy world where bad things happen to those who are hurting us. Our lower mind creates a world in which our negative emotions are justified. It is our right to feel these things. It is our right to place ourselves in a prison of negative emotions. If we keep on insisting on this right, then we may create a hardwired network in our brain that perpetuates these emotions. Our desire to escape discomfort grooves a thinking pattern that creates more discomfort. We become trapped in our lower mind.

Instead of pursuing these escape routes, we must learn to stop and experience our negative feelings—and manage them without pursuing an unhealthy diversion. So let's step back for a moment and consider some of the many different ways that people can think about the world around them and the world within them. Consider the following:

- Positive versus negative
- Learning mode versus knowing mode
- Growth mindset versus fixed mindset
- Other-focused versus self-focused
- Present-focused versus past- or future-focused

Learning mode describes people who are always trying to grow and learn. They're open to new things and they don't assume they know everything. They're ready to engage with a problem in order to learn more. They don't spend a lot of time measuring themselves against other people; they're interested in *learning* from other people.

Compare that to knowing mode, in which people feel they already know the answers and don't need to learn more. They feel they're right, while others are wrong. They know best, while others don't. Knowing mode is a closed mindset in which people, by and large, do not grow.

Then there's the growth mindset versus the fixed mindset, as explained in more detail in the great book *Mindset* by Carol Dweck. The growth mindset is similar to learning mode. In a growth mindset, people are embracing challenges, they're open to new learning, and they perceive stressors as something to work through. They don't look at failure as failure, but rather as an opportunity to learn and improve. People in the growth mindset tend to build other people up and tend to be very successful in whatever area of life they find themselves. They tend to have positive relationships.

That's in contrast to fixed-mindset individuals, who see their own capacity and the capacity of others as immutable. They think intelligence is fixed. They view failure as final. Interestingly, people with the fixed mindset often end up cheating, because their identities are so dependent on specific outcomes. They tend not to be supportive of others, and they tend to be very self-absorbed and focused on reputation.

Then there's other-focused as opposed to self-focused. People who are other-focused tend to live their lives in service to others and to view others as more important than themselves. They look at the world from the perspective of what they can do to benefit those around them. They help others realize their full potential. In contrast, as you'd expect, people who are self-focused tend to live life according to their own desires. They also tend to inflate their own egos to feel better about themselves.

Finally, there's present-focused versus past- or future-focused. Even though there are countless clichés about living in the present, most of us don't do a good job of it. In fact, many of us do a really bad job of staying in the present. We're dominated by our past and future. We tend to spend a huge amount of time ruminating about the past, feeling guilty, ashamed, or angry. We constantly relive the past in our own minds, even though the past is past, and nothing will ever change it. It exists now only in the form of memory, which is nothing more than chemicals and connections stored in our brains. That's the only place the past exists. And yet we give over so many of our present moments to dwelling in that disappeared past.

We do the same with the future. We worry about the future in ways large and small—and the vast majority of things we worry about never actually come to pass. We worry about uncertainty. Perhaps your job is uncertain, or a loved one is ill. Those are genuinely concerning, of course, and yet we can't always know what will happen. So we worry about what *might* happen. We also listen to and read sensationalized news about what's happening all around the world, and we worry about events that are affecting people we've never met. We might worry about the much-hyped collapse of our economy or political system. We also might ruminate on the things we *want* to happen—whether for our loved ones or ourselves, whether realistic or not.

Everyone knows we can't accurately predict the future. In fact, the vast majority of the things we worry about, *and* the things we hope for, won't actually take place, at least not as we imagine them. Yet we become completely engrossed in the stories of our minds. We *believe* that our stories are true.

And we do all of that at the expense of the present. If we live our lives focused on the past or the future, what we're actually doing is giving up the only moment that's real: this moment, right now. It's the only moment that matters. It's the only moment that you can count on and the only one you can control. And for the rest of your life, there will be a sequence of present moments, and then your life will end. And at that point, you either will have lived your life in those present moments, or you will have given them up to the past or future—in which case you've lived no life at all.

All the forces around us are conspiring to keep us from the present. All the social media, all the pop-up advertising on your computer screen, all the emails that aren't about important things, all the notifications coming through your phone, all the sensationalized news reports—all of those are taking you from your present moment. They're taking you away from the one real thing you have.

In contrast, when you actually focus on the present, you have control in a way that you never did before. Of course, you don't have control over the events of the world, or even many of the events of your own life. But you now have the ability to choose your response to the circumstances and challenges before you.

You can choose positivity and growth and learning, rather than a negative or closed approach. You can choose to direct your energies toward your cherished purpose in life—whether that's your family, your profession, your community, your health, or any of a million other purposes and goals. In fact, the only time that you *do* want to focus on the future is when you're developing goals and plans regarding your genuine purpose in this world and how you hope to realize that purpose in the greatest possible way. That's a future worth living in—briefly. Then bring yourself back into the present, so that you can use this moment in a way that's in alignment with your larger purpose.

When you've shifted your orientation from past- and future-focused to present-focused, it will allow you to make the best choices for your health. From breathing, hydrating, and eating to how you hold your body and how you manage your emotions, you'll have the awareness and motivation necessary for making the best choices—so you'll have the energy you want and need for a life of meaning and purpose.

All of us need to feel that sense of meaning in our lives. Some mind states—those that are positive, conducive to learning and growth, and present- and other-focused—help us to fulfill that essential need. The psychologist Martin Seligman uses an acronym, PERMA, to summarize some of the core needs, including meaning, that must be fulfilled in order for us to feel a sense of well-being.

PERMA stands for:

- Positive Emotion
- Engagement
- Positive Relationships
- Meaning
- Accomplishment

Everyone needs these things to feel a sense of well-being. Positive emotions include things like love, hope, and peacefulness. Engagement refers to a sense of being immersed in something that you find absorbing, that makes your brain thrive, and that allows you to lose a sense of yourself. Positive relationships refer to having strong, meaningful connections to others. Meaning is, of course, that sense of purpose. And accomplishment refers to feeling a sense of progress toward goals.

Everyone needs these five areas of PERMA. If you'd like, you can use Martin Seligman's online resources, available at www.authentichappiness.sas.upenn.edu, to do an inventory that will help you understand any areas where you might be lacking and thus will help you develop a greater sense of well-being. Those with a strong sense of overall well-being are more likely to choose habits that increase their well-being—in other words, well-being is self-perpetuating.

It's important to recognize that all of us are a mix of these different mindsets and qualities. All of us are both positive and negative, at different times and in different moments. We're all growth and fixed. We're all selfish, but also serving others. And all of us, at some point, give away our present moment to the past or future. But the intention here is to help you move toward a mindset that will give you a greater sense of well-being, and thereby encourage you to make the right choices and habits for your health—and for your deeper purpose.

If I were to pick one mindset quality for you to focus on, it would be gratitude. A grateful mindset is a powerful catalyst for positivity. Try to start each day reflecting on what you are grateful for. Focusing on the good things in your life will move you from a negative emotional state to a positive emotional state. Studies have shown that even if you cannot think of one thing you are grateful for, just trying to find something to be grateful for will initiate a positive emotional response. Gratitude is a powerful thinking habit.

TAKE NOTE OF YOUR HABITS—AND BEGIN MOVING IN A NEW DIRECTION

You now understand that many of your habits are rooted in memories or events that happened a long time ago and were probably beyond your control. You also now know that you have the ability to change your habits, thanks to the power of your brain.

Right there, you've taken a couple important steps forward. One key to the process of finding good health is recognizing that just about everything you do is a habit, and that you have the power to change. It's also helpful to understand, as best you can, the reasons behind your habits. Remember the habit loop I mentioned earlier in the chapter. Your brain has been conditioned to respond to certain events with specific behaviors because of some reward that follows that behavior. Understanding your habit loop will help you to understand yourself, and that will help you in your process of change.

That's why it's essential that you start to take note of your habits—I mean, literally write them down. This is *very* important. Start to take an inventory. What are you doing first thing in the morning? How are you envisioning your workday and your responsibilities? How are you feeding yourself? How are you breathing? Are you aware of your physical body? Are you feeling stressed, and if so, are you aware of your stressors? Are you thinking about what you genuinely desire before you make choices? Which of your daily habits take you closer to your desires, and which move you further away?

Journaling in this way is invaluable. It forces you to stop and think about what you're doing, and the recorded notes allow you to see patterns that you wouldn't otherwise recognize. That gives you the opportunity to engage more mindfully in the choices you're making all day, every day. Then you can evaluate your habits to see if they're worth keeping. If you decide that some of them need to change, you can proceed by making a plan and then noting your progress, as well as setbacks, as you move forward.

You'll be tempted to judge yourself during this process. You might even be inclined to judge yourself harshly—because it's hard to change habits. You won't succeed right away, which is likely to trigger an onslaught of negative emotions. But consider this: the failures and successes that you experience are part of a crucial process in which you uncover your subconscious drivers.

You'll see which habits are hardest to break and which are the easiest. Over time, that awareness helps you to gain mastery over your habits. If you succeeded right away, you wouldn't learn the things about yourself that you really need to know as part of your larger shift toward good health. So when you start to feel judgmental toward yourself, try to redirect your attention back to the process itself.

Most of all, it's important to remember that you *are* capable of changing in the ways that you desire. You've really got to trust that. You have to trust in your ability to overcome your past traumas and failures and to put your fears about the future to rest. That's the route to authentic well-being and to engagement in the present moment—the only moment you have.

STEP INTO THE CONSULTATION ROOM

Let's apply all this material about thinking and habits to a setting that's likely very familiar to you: a doctor's office. Let's say that you've come in to my office with a specific set of concerns, including fatigue, weight gain, body pain, and low-level depression. You've done some reading online and you tell me that you think you may have a hormonal problem.

I interview you about your symptoms. I ask questions regarding your medical history, your family history, and your medications. Do you smoke? Do you drink, and if so, how much? We draw blood and run lab tests.

But your tests come back negative; there's nothing to suggest that your symptoms are the result of any disease. You're normal—except for the painful symptoms that continue to plague you.

That might not sound like good news, but it is. Everything that's happening to you is reversible. You have the power to change the things that are making you sick.

In the consultation room, our conversation now moves in a different direction. I ask about your habits and we begin discussing your diet, your sleep patterns, your emotional health, and how physically active you are. We do this because identifying your existing habits is a crucial first step on the road to developing new, healthier habits.

You tell me that you're not sleeping soundly, that you often feel quite stressed, and that you generally don't exercise much. On the question of diet, you say that you don't eat too well. All of this is consistent with the experience and habits of many of the patients who walk through my office door each day.

Next, we try to understand what's behind your current habits. You've told me that you had a burger and fries for dinner last night, so I ask, "What was happening for you when you decided to eat that particular meal?" I'm simply trying to understand what's driving your choices. Until you understand the behavioral causes behind your choices, it will be extremely hard or even impossible for you to change habits.

When I ask about the burger and fries, you think for a minute and then say simply that you weren't thinking a whole lot about that particular meal choice; you were busy, you didn't have a lot of time, and that's a go-to meal. Plus, it tastes good.

So now we've begun to review your habits, and we've started to reveal what's behind them. Next we're going to start to identify what you really want for yourself.

"I want to be healthy," you tell me. "I want to have energy and to just feel good in my body."

"Okay, let's go back to your habits and choices," I say. We review the habits that you've just described to me. "Do you truly desire to be well?"

"I *do* want to be well," you reply. You also acknowledge that many of your habits aren't consistent with that desire; over time, you've been conditioned to make choices that take you *away* from what you want for yourself, rather than closer to it.

At this point in the exam, I write you an initial prescription. From the material in this chapter, you know that moving toward better health will involve changing your thinking. And that's why I start out by prescribing you three tools that will help you equip your brain to gain a greater mastery over your choices:

- Engage in a minimum of fifteen minutes of daily aerobic activity. (Increase time if desired, but do a minimum of fifteen minutes.) This can be in any form you want: walking, swimming, biking, dancing, skipping rope, you name it. You just have to get your heart rate up.

- Do a set of daily exercises to help sharpen your focus. Examples of these exercises can be found at the end of this chapter. They involve just breathing and then focusing and holding your attention, and simply practicing this as a habit.

- Identify and pursue something that you've wanted to try but haven't. It could be pottery, music, art, reading a book on an unfamiliar topic, or even re-learning math. It can be anything that will create a novel learning experience—because doing so will help you get your brain into shape.

This prescription actually doesn't sound too difficult to you. Basically, you've got to start doing the three things that enhance neuroplasticity—aerobic exercise, techniques for sharpening mental focus, and new learning experiences— and you've got to start tracking your habits. That's it! You agree to start immediately, and we decide that you'll come back to my office in a few weeks.

Now, before we move on to the next chapter, I have to make one final note. You may be tempted to discount all of this stuff about thinking and habit. You may have come to this book hoping for a simple diet plan or exercise recommendations, and you may be tempted just to skip to the later chapters instead of starting out with your thinking. But trust me on this: the later chapters won't help you unless you're focused on thinking and habit. At its core, each chapter of this book is about habit—and about the power of the brain to create new habits.

It's also possible that your habits may be rooted in a painful past that's simply too difficult for you to approach without professional help. If you think that might be the case, I strongly recommend that you meet with a behavioral therapist and begin to explore this subject in a dedicated way. This recommendation is something that we'll return to in later chapters.

FINAL POINTS

- You must desire your own health and vitality. Only you can want it for yourself. Desire is foundational to any achievement.

- You must know your own story: why you think, emote, and act the way you do.

- You must take an inventory and track your habits. Are your habits taking you toward what you want for yourself, or further away from it?

- You must believe in your ability to change and cultivate a growth mindset that is focused and grounded in positivity.

EXERCISES TO SHARPEN YOUR FOCUS

The following exercises will strengthen your higher mind and potentiate change. You do not need to do them all. Just pick one or two and practice them regularly. Start with five minutes daily and build from there. Keep things simple and be patient with yourself. You must exercise your higher mind for it to work for you.

Focus Drill: Take deep relaxing breaths and calm your mind. Pick out a spot on a wall or, if you're outside, on a distant object. Focus on that spot for thirty seconds. Then move your focus to a spot in the center of the room or in the center of space about twelve feet away from you. This will literally be at the center of the volume of the room; it will be more difficult than you think. Focus on this spot for thirty seconds. Now move your focus to about twelve inches front in front of you, as if you were looking at a book or a tablet. Focus on that spot for thirty seconds. Now move back to the center of the room for thirty seconds, and then back to the distant spot for thirty seconds. Repeat this for up to five minutes—or longer, if you're able. This exercise will greatly enhance your focus. It's also perfect to do right before you need to work on a project or focus intently on something that you need to get done. Even doing this drill for one minute can be helpful.

Insight Meditation: Sit comfortably. Begin to breathe deeply and to count your breaths. Calm your mind. Pick an internal quality or value that you either possess or that you want to possess, such as courage, or the

Golden Rule. Begin to focus and examine this quality. Your goal is to look into your own beliefs and values, to understand them better. If a feeling of judgment arises as you do this (about yourself, or about the quality you're examining, or about this meditation exercise, or anything else) try to just notice the judgment and then dismiss it without getting caught up in it. You're seeking to strengthen and deepen the beliefs and values that are consistent with the person you want to be in the world.

When reflecting on your beliefs and values in this way, it can be helpful to look at them from multiple perspectives to better understand them. For example, if you're focusing on the Golden Rule, you can consider it from the perspective of the person who is acting and the person on the receiving end of the action. Through this process, you're trying to make your beliefs and your values truly your own and to understand them fully. If possible, engage in this exercise for fifteen minutes. (Even five minutes will be useful.)

Contemplation: Pick an external concept or circumstance about which you want to deepen your understanding—such as a work of art or even a beautiful sunset. Contemplate it from multiple perspectives. If you're focusing on the sunset, consider its different strands of color, and the way it looks in the sky as well as the way it changes the light around you, or any other dimensions that you might observe. The idea is to contemplate deeply whatever you have chosen in a manner that stimulates your desire for a positive attribute. Contemplating the sunset may stimulate your desire for peace or for beauty. If possible, engage in this exercise for fifteen minutes. (Even five minutes will be useful.)

Positive Visualization: Picture what you desire for this day or for your future. Visualize it in a very detailed manner. Feel it, see it, and experience it. Positively visualize how it would feel to arrive at your desired future. Picture what it takes to get to these desired results. If possible, engage in this exercise for fifteen minutes. (Even five minutes will be useful.)

Recapitulation: Revisit past experiences in order to understand them better. Sitting peacefully, begin to recall and consider challenging periods earlier in your life. Try to study these difficult periods as if you were an outsider. Your goal is to better understand yourself and the challenges that you've faced, as well as the ways that you've responded to those challenges. Recapitulation can serve to expose limiting beliefs or negative thinking patterns that may have plagued you throughout your life. What's more, you will then have the opportunity to use your new understanding to create a better future, by observing ways in which you might want to change your thinking patterns moving forward. If possible, engage in this exercise for fifteen minutes. (Even five minutes will be useful.)

Gratitude Exercise: Try to start every day by thinking of 3 things you are grateful for. Just think about those things and how glad you are for them. Spend a few minutes thinking about everything you are grateful for. Try to do this at the end of your day as well. Try to bookend your day with a mindset of gratitude.

ADDITIONAL RESOURCES

- *The 7 Habits of Highly Effective People*, by Stephen Covey
- *The Power of Full Engagement: Managing Energy, Not Time, Is the Key to High Performance and Personal Renewal* by Jim Loehr and Tony Schwartz
- *Mindset,* by Carol Dweck
- *The Power of Habit,* by Charles Duhigg
- *Switch: How to Change Things When Change is Hard,* by Chip Heath and Dan Heath
- Our resources at www.healthshepherds.com

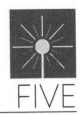

FIVE

Changing Habits by Doing

*This chapter provides a simple process for developing self-control
and increasing willpower. You will learn how to control and redirect
powerful cravings so that you can make choices consistent with your
desire for genuine health. You can condition your brain to choose
health, once you know how. Willpower is a skill that can be developed.*

SOMETHING STRANGE AND powerful has been affecting our brains
over the past several decades, and until recently, it was poorly understood.
But now we have reliable scientific evidence to better understand how our
modern world affects some of our most basic neural wiring.

Most likely you're familiar with the concept of "fight or flight." That's
our physiological response to a perceived threat, and it's our body's way of
preparing either to engage or flee. The fight-or-flight reaction also triggers
the release of stress hormones in the body—and it affects the way the
brain functions.

For the sake of simplifying, let's say that the human brain has three
major parts to it. The first is the most primitive part, and it governs your
fight-or-flight response. The purpose of this region is to alert you to threats
and then prompt you to take action. No higher-level thinking or reasoning
happens in this area of the brain; the impulses here are essentially on auto-
pilot, and the physiological responses they initiate are reflexive.

The second part of your brain is more advanced than the first. Consider this your mammalian brain. This is the region responsible for memories,

habits, and emotions (I'm simplifying, of course, but this is enough to give you a sense of how things work). This region also handles some of your thinking and decision-making.

Finally, there's the most advanced area of the human brain, which includes your prefrontal cortex. This is your higher mind, the place where the brain integrates functions and impulses from the other two areas and engages in complex reasoning. You could say that this is where the magic happens. The prefrontal cortex sets humans apart from other species.

When the prefrontal cortex is activated and influencing our overall brain function, we tend to feel in control of our emotions. We are able to think in an integrated manner; we're able to form the right responses to the situations in front of us. We're able to do this because we have greater willpower and self-control when the prefrontal cortex is functioning properly. But the opposite is also true: when the prefrontal cortex isn't fully functional, our ability to govern our behaviors declines. Our behavior becomes very predictable.

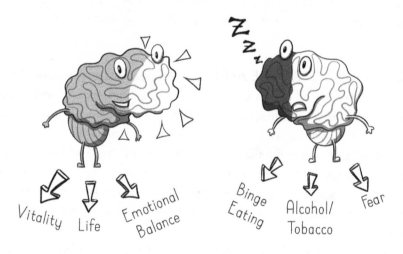

Vitality   Life   Emotional Balance   Binge Eating   Alcohol/ Tobacco   Fear

Now consider the fact that stress tends to foster a sense of fear. That is, when you're stressed, it tends to manifest not only as angst but also, very often, as fear and panic. The fear and panic then trigger your primitive brain—because your brain thinks you're in danger. That turns on your fight-or-flight response.

When your fight-or-flight response is activated, it *directly inhibits* normal functioning in the prefrontal cortex. There's a biological reason for this. If you're facing a genuine threat to your safety, you no longer need to spend time planning or thinking; it's time for action. So your fight-or-flight system is designed to *turn off* your prefrontal cortex and get you moving. Once again, I am over simplifying the process, but the overall idea is correct.

You've probably noticed that you tend not to think as clearly when you're feeling stressed out. You also may have noticed that your self-control declines and that you tend to give in to your less desirable habits. Now you understand part of the reason: your higher mind switches off when you feel the fear and panic that often accompany stress. When stressed out, we're more likely to drink, gamble, overeat, or park ourselves in front of the television. We seem to have little self-control in these times *because we really do have less self-control*; our ability to control our impulses during stressful times actually drops.

From a biological perspective, it makes sense that our thinking and reasoning mind switches off when we face danger. But this has terrible consequences in our modern world. Today, our fight-or-flight reaction is continuously triggered by stimuli that are no real threat to us at all. There are scary news reports, worrisome emails, and upsetting tweets. There are arguments and controversies posted every instant on Facebook.

This constitutes a continual barrage of fear-inducing stimuli on our brains. We feel constantly stressed, and that stress triggers our fight-or-flight response, which in turn inhibits the one area of our brain that we need the most: our higher mind.

If you actually stop and examine the situations that make you stressed, you'll very often discover that they're not worth being anxious about. (We'll talk a lot about this type of awareness in the next chapter.) Indeed, we don't need our fight-or-flight response in order to deal with most of the scary things we face in our modern world; we need our *thinking* brain. We need to be able to make measured decisions—including the decision not to get stressed out.

DOPAMINE AND THE POWER OF CRAVINGS

The power of dopamine complicates matters even more. Laboratory rats have been found to repeat behaviors when those behaviors stimulate a particular area of the brain. Scientists used to believe that these rats were experiencing a pleasurable sensation in that brain region. Thus, they initially called that part of the brain "the pleasure center."

But it was later discovered that they had not interpreted correctly the feeling those rats were experiencing; the rats weren't experiencing pleasure, but rather the *anticipation* of pleasure. In other words, they were experiencing a craving. And this sensation of craving was found to be specifically associated with a neurotransmitter called dopamine. The release of dopamine was associated with strong cravings and the anticipation of pleasure, but no real satisfaction. That's why the rats kept engaging in the same behavior: they sought a sense of pleasure that kept diminishing.

This happens in the human brain, too. We feel powerful cravings for substances and activities that are associated with the release of dopamine. But dopamine-fueled cravings tend not to bring any persistent satisfaction. And not only do we fail to experience real pleasure from them, but they tend to be associated with *even greater stress*. Unfortunately, when we experience a dopamine-fueled craving, we often can't control ourselves.

This area of our brain is often referred to as the reward system. It serves a purpose. We are designed to experience pleasure with activities that promote our survival and the future of our species. We do actually experience pleasure when we eat certain foods and engage in certain activities. Dopamine serves as a motivator. It stimulates desire and motivates us to satisfy our cravings. Once we encounter a substance or activity that activates our reward system, we release chemicals in our brain called endogenous opiate peptides or EOP's. These do provide a brief experience of pleasure, and we are designed to remember what caused this pleasure. We can then repeat this behavior as the opportunity arises.

This system works fine as long as the substances and behaviors that produce the pleasure are only available in limited quantities and infrequently. When activators of the reward system (drugs, alcohol, pornography, gambling, sugar, fat, video games, etc.) are super concentrated and readily available, we lose control of our behavioral responses. We cannot control our use of these substances, and eventually, they no longer even provide pleasure. They just make us sick and depressed. However, we cannot seem to stop using whatever it is we crave.

Let's take this one step further. As the power of dopamine has become more widely understood in our modern world, companies have *intentionally exploited it* as a means of marketing and selling us more stuff. Major corporations actually employ behavioral psychologists and neuroscientists to figure out how to trigger that dopamine pathway so that we'll repeatedly buy their products or pursue whatever they're offering. This phenomenon is particularly well known in the video game industry, but it also applies to food companies and many other sectors. Essentially, our brains are being manipulated—just like those of rats in a lab.

Pain and pleasure are meant to draw our attention to what created that particular feeling. These feelings are supposed to give us information about what actions or behaviors we need to undertake. The brain, like the rest of our body, moves toward homeostasis, the tendency to find balance when facing internal and external changes. I like the way Dr. Anna Lembke, the head of addiction medicine at Stanford University, describes this phenomenon: "There is no free lunch in the brain."

Dr. Lembke describes pain and pleasure as a seesaw. Push on one, the brain will adjust toward the other. Opioids, alcohol, amphetamines, and other addictive substances that push hard on the pleasure side will produce an increase on the pain side. But if you engage in strenuous activities that may cause pain, the brain will regulate upward the communication of pleasure. That's why we feel good after a great workout. We aren't supposed to short-circuit the pleasure pathway with medications, addictive foods, addictive tech, or any other direct stimulator of dopamine. We're supposed to get our dopamine naturally.

Though we won't get into the details of brain chemistry, research by the American Psychological Association has figured out which specific activities are associated with dopamine-fueled cravings, greater stress, and no real satisfaction.

Activities associated with the *anticipation* of pleasure, but no genuine pleasure at all, include:

- binge eating
- drinking alcohol in excess
- binge shopping
- using tobacco
- watching stress inducing television programs

- surfing the web
- playing video games (specifically those designed to be addictive)
- gambling
- using addictive substances such as opioids and other drugs

Though we tend to experience overpowering cravings for these activities, performing the activities doesn't translate into any real satisfaction. These activities also have been found to be the *least* effective for coping with stress—even though they are precisely the activities we tend to pursue when we *are* stressed. Why? In part, it's because the dopamine-fueled craving is powerful, and in part it's because our self-control is compromised. The release of hormones associated with these cravings then facilitates still higher levels of stress—and, very often, shame and guilt, too.

There's a vicious cycle at work here. When we feel stressed, that makes us fearful, which turns off our higher mind. At the same time, we feel a craving for unhealthy behaviors. Our self-control is inhibited, so we cave in to those cravings. Afterward, we feel guilty for doing so, which makes us feel even more stressed. Then the cycle repeats. And the more you engage in this cycle, the more completely your higher mind switches off and the more completely you'll feel controlled by the cravings.

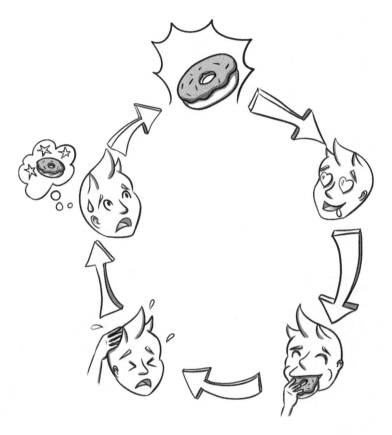

But the American Psychological Association has also studied which activities offer genuine satisfaction and a pathway to a sustained sense of well-being. Activities associated with sustained improvements in long-term well-being include:

- meditation
- exercise or playing sports
- sleep
- relaxation (not turning on the television, but simply relaxing and letting your brain rest)
- attending religious ceremonies
- praying
- reading

- listening to music
- doing yoga
- engaging in creative hobbies
- spending time with loved ones

According to the research, these activities prompt restorative responses in the body and slow down the production of stress hormones. These activities increase serotonin, oxytocin, and other feel-good neurochemicals in your brain. This leads to a sustained sense of well-being. And that is important news—because now that you understand a bit about what's happening in your brain, you can *do* something about it.

DOING: THE TRICK TO OVERPOWERING YOUR CRAVINGS

By their very nature, cravings are extremely hard to resist. When the dopamine transmitter is activated, there's a surge of adrenaline, and it often feels exciting. In that moment, when you feel the power of the craving, the anticipation of having it satisfied seems more pleasurable than almost anything else—and certainly more pleasurable than, for instance, meditating or exercising.

What's more, because our stress response has been activated, our higher mind has turned off. That's the part of the brain that could step out of the situation and decide, for instance, that drinking or binge eating or watching television might not be the best course of action.

After all, your higher mind is the part of you that knows what you *truly* desire for yourself. You truly desire health—but in the moment of the craving, with your higher mind switched off, that larger desire seems secondary to the anticipated pleasure of giving in to the craving.

So here's a powerful, evidence-based approach to addressing the problem.

The next time you feel yourself beginning to crave a substance or activity that you know is unhealthy—whether it is junk food or alcohol or television or something else—*wait ten minutes*. And in those ten minutes, select an activity from the second list, above. Go for a walk or talk to a loved one or just relax quietly. Research suggests that if you engage in one of these healthy activities for ten minutes or more—instead of giving in to a craving— more often than not, the power of the craving will diminish.

If you follow this approach, you will have taken two important steps toward better health. The first step was to resist your craving, and the second was to engage in a positive activity that contributes to your long-term health.

Here's a step-by-step breakdown. When you start to feel a craving:

1. Look at the clock. Tell yourself that you only have to wait ten minutes before deciding on how to respond to whatever you are craving.

2. Choose a healthy activity from the second list above. Engage in that activity for at least ten minutes.

3. Take a minute to assess how you're feeling in body and mind. Are you still experiencing the craving? Has it gotten weaker? Consider continuing the healthy activity you've started rather than giving in to the craving. Can you do it?

Interestingly, there's a lot of evidence to show that when people pay close attention to how they're feeling during a craving, the craving actually starts to reduce. That is, just paying attention and becoming aware of what you're feeling is a lot of the battle.

We're going to discuss this idea of awareness a lot more in the coming chapters, including Chapter Seven, when we'll talk about eating habits and the power of slowing down while eating. As it turns out, research indicates that when people really pay attention to what they're eating and how it makes them feel, they very often discover that the most tantalizing junk foods aren't truly satisfying. Often those foods look and smell better than they actually taste. But when we binge eat, we tend to eat so much food, so quickly, that we hardly taste any of it—and thus we don't even realize that we don't feel satisfied.

Slowing down and becoming aware of what's happening will also train your brain in new habits and patterns. Right now your brain may be accustomed to feeling the surge of hormones associated with binging. Simply slowing down and paying attention to what you're doing, and how it feels, reduces the hormones and stress associated with craving and binging.

Awareness also helps to foster long-term resilience and self-control. As you start to slow down and delay that indulgence, you actually teach your brain to adjust its expectations, so that when a craving comes on, it's no longer such an intense surge of hormones. That, in turn, allows your higher brain to switch on again. And that allows you to consider and then pursue what you truly want for yourself.

You could call this a strange moment in human history. As far as we know, it's unprecedented in our history that our dopamine pathways could be triggered so many times a day by people we don't even know—because strangers now have direct access to our brains through our television and devices. The ability to market directly to consumers is unique to our modern world. We've always been susceptible to snake oil, but never in history has snake oil been sold to us all day long from so many directions and then delivered almost instantaneously.

And that's why it's essential that we start waking up. We have to acknowledge that powerful forces are conditioning our brains and behaviors and that our desires are being manipulated. Think for a moment about the things you tend to crave throughout your day. How many of those things are good for you? How many are destructive to your health *and* translate into profit for someone else?

We have to wake up to the reality that our devices and our televisions and our data plans rarely give us any real satisfaction and that they give us, instead, manufactured lives in which we are unhealthy and unhappy. Never before in history has so much money been made by selling us dopamine-boosting products that leave us feeling empty and sick.

To recover the health that you want for yourself, you will have to reject much of the power of the modern marketplace. You will have to come to your own understanding about the real sources of well-being. You cannot buy well-being, but you can earn it.

DEALING WITH GUILT AND OTHER STRESSFUL THOUGHTS

No one's perfect. No matter how good your intentions or determination, there will undoubtedly be times when you give in to your cravings.

What's deeply important is that you don't berate yourself afterward. Indeed, we're often flooded with feelings of shame and guilt at those times. But the self-criticism and negativity actually make us feel more stressed—and that translates into still more destructive behaviors.

It's essential that we instead choose to practice self-forgiveness. This is a time to be kind to ourselves. We must recognize that all of us have shortcomings, all of us are going to fail sometimes, and it's the journey that defines who we are. This quest is easier said than done. So here's a brief guideline for battling self-criticism.

The goal is to forgive yourself as quickly as possible when you find that you're engaging in an unhealthy behavior. Even in the moment that you're eating an unhealthy food, for instance, remind yourself that we all have shortcomings. If possible, offer yourself forgiveness out loud: "I forgive myself." This is actually very important; dwelling in self-criticism will only increase your stress responses. By firmly offering forgiveness in the moment, you can help get yourself back on a positive pathway.

Immediately forgiving yourself will *reduce* stress and, as you now know, lowering stress will help to reactivate your higher mind. Then you can once again remember what you really want—you really want *health*—and then make better decisions accordingly.

If you, like so many of us, find it extremely difficult to forgive yourself, here's an exercise to try.

When you've binged on unhealthy foods or otherwise abandoned your plan for better health, stop for a moment and pretend that the person in question isn't you. Instead, imagine that this person is a friend of yours. This friend has been sick for some time and is really trying to get better—but he or she has just fallen off the wagon.

What would you say to such friends? I'm guessing you wouldn't berate them. Instead, you'd likely feel compassion for them. You would look at the bigger picture and see that they're really trying to improve, and that surely they will make progress, and that it's okay that they've fallen off the wagon in this particular moment. You would offer your encouragement and support. You would probably say that you believe in them and that you know they can do this.

Then step back. Tell yourself that you are deserving of the same encouragement and support that you would give to that friend. In other words, it's time to *become that friend to yourself*. Don't give in to the feelings of shame.

Another strategy is a means of dealing directly with stressful or self-critical thoughts when they arise. It's important that you don't try to suppress those thoughts. Imagine if I said to you, "Don't think about a red puppy." After that, of course, you wouldn't be able to stop thinking about a red puppy. Indeed, evidence shows that our attempts to suppress thoughts simply don't work—in fact, they simply cause us to dwell on the very things we're trying to avoid.

Instead—strange as it may sound—the best strategy is acceptance. We can't control most of our thoughts, so it's important just to accept that some of our thoughts are unproductive or painful. Make it your goal to just sit with that discomfort rather than try to avoid it. This won't necessarily be easy, but here's a strategy to use when you need it.

When you begin to experience an uncomfortable thought—whether it's anxiety about something that happened at work, or your worries about what's going on in this country, or a sense of craving for an unhealthy activity—the best approach is to do some deep breathing. (Specific guidelines for controlled breathing are in the next chapter.)

Start by taking a few deep breaths. As you occupy this breathing space for a few minutes, you will actually have the chance to see your thoughts for what they are. Maybe you can actually picture them as clouds floating by. Then try to regard them the way you would real clouds in the sky overhead: "Isn't that cloud interesting? Look at its strange shape. That's funny." You can even pretend that your breathing is the wind that blows the clouds away.

By slowing down and breathing deeply in this way, you counteract your stress responses and allow your higher mind to switch on. You've turned off your fight-or-flight response. And now you have the chance to use your higher mind to redirect your thoughts. If you're experiencing a craving, now is the time to refocus on what you actually want for yourself.

As you begin to experiment with this approach, you might find that this isn't enough to keep you from giving in to your stress-induced cravings or stressful thoughts. Don't worry. Remind yourself that there's nothing wrong with you for having those thoughts or cravings. And as long as you continue to experiment with this process of thought acceptance, you will absolutely make progress over time. I can promise you that.

If you stick with this, you will develop greater resilience. Through controlled breathing and through naming and accepting your uncomfortable thoughts, you'll build the self-control necessary for resisting unhealthy behaviors. You cannot control your thoughts, but you can begin to control the behaviors those thoughts produce. Over time, as they have less influence, the thoughts will occur less frequently.

FOSTERING HOPE—INSTEAD OF FALSE HOPE

It's important to distinguish between genuine hope and something called "false hope syndrome." False hope syndrome is when you resolve to do something in order to make you feel better in the moment.

Let's say that you've been binging on unhealthy foods. In a surge of shame, you resolve that you're going to start a new diet—on Monday. Then you picture yourself on this new diet, and you picture yourself losing weight. Well, that act of simply imagining yourself making a change actually gives you a little dopamine burst and a momentary sense of euphoria. Suddenly, you feel good about the new diet that you're going to start on Monday, and how much weight you're going to lose as a result of it. Perhaps you start searching the Internet for programs or devices that will help you. That, too, gives you a little dopamine surge. So now you're feeling good—just by imagining this stuff.

But this behavior is actually an attempt to fix your momentary guilty *feeling* and not your underlying bad *habits*. The sense of euphoria that accompanies a decision to change—without actually making any change—pulls you out of the despair. And if all you really wanted was to stop feeling bad in the moment, rather than to create lasting change for yourself, then you have solved your problem. Now you can actually forget about the decision to change in the future, which allows you to fall right back in with the very habits that triggered the shame and despair in the first place.

One way of addressing this problem is through something called "future continuity." Essentially, it's important that you foster a sense of connection between yourself at this point in time and yourself in the future. That might seem obvious, but we humans often act in ways that discount our future selves. So it's deeply important that you orient yourself toward connecting with your future and the things you really want for yourself. A strong sense of future continuity is associated with much greater self-control. You have to be deeply connected to your future self and remember that you will be living in this same body decades from now. Most individuals have future continuity when it involves their fiscal future or profession, but we seem to be missing it when it comes to our health. If you provide your future self an unhealthy body, all of your other planning will not matter quite as much.

In Chapter Ten, we're going to talk about this a lot more. We're going to get into the question of your life's purpose, and you'll have exercises to help you visualize the future you want. It's very important to do the exercises; they'll help you orient your behaviors in the present moment with your genuine hope for the future.

HOW HE CHANGED HIS HEALTH BY *DOING*

I'd like to tell you about my patient James, who served in the Marines as a young person and then started his own business. Eventually, he transitioned into a job in which he works at a desk every day. Over the next several years after taking the desk job, he gained about thirty pounds, and he also ended up on medications for his blood pressure, cholesterol, and reflux. When he came in for his regular check-up appointment, he was usually very energetic and positive, and I always enjoyed seeing him.

But at one of his annual check-ups, I walked into the exam room and saw that he was different. He looked angry. He immediately asked my opinion about a recent public-health issue that he was very worried about. I listened to him for a while, and then I realized the he had been listening to inflammatory news reporting and that he was missing key pieces of the story. As I began to flesh out the whole story for him, his demeanor changed.

Finally, he looked up at me and said, "I've got to stop watching these news channels."

I encouraged him to do just that. I explained how modern TV news is designed to trigger fear, stress, and a craving to keep watching and to keep checking back for updates. I explained how, regardless of the political bias represented, the modern-day news cycles were primarily focused on increasing their viewership in order to increase the wealth of the networks. James agreed with me, and we wrapped up the visit by going through our typical process for a check-up.

After that, I didn't see James for fifteen months—which was unusual, because he normally came in annually for refills on his medications. When he finally did come back to my office, he looked quite different. In fact, he looked younger and leaner and happier.

"How does my blood work look, Doc?" he asked.

I opened his results—and, as it turned out, they looked excellent. His blood pressure was also normal, and I noticed that he had lost about thirty pounds. He'd also stopped needing his medications.

"You look just great, James," I said, putting away the paperwork. "How did you do it?"

He told me that after our last visit, he had stopped watching cable news. Instead, in the evenings, he would exercise with his son or engage in other hobbies. He said it had been challenging at first. He'd felt a strong craving to watch the news, that he might be missing something important.

"But whenever I felt that feeling coming on, I would just go to the garage and start working out," he said.

Soon he had no desire to turn on the television. He explained that while he was still affirmed in his political views, he no longer felt angry. He said he found himself less judgmental of others and more compassionate. Before long, he had no desire for the news at all; he just wanted to be with his family and to be physically active.

It's amazing how much this one change accomplished for James. He turned off the TV and substituted exercise in its place. His brain had been conditioned to crave the news, so this took a lot of effort on his part. But because he had a deep desire to feel healthier—and especially to feel less stressed and less angry—he succeeded. In the process, he also reversed three chronic conditions that he'd previously needed medications to control.

Suddenly, he found himself in great health, in both mind and body.

STEP INTO THE CONSULTATION ROOM

This time, when you come in to my office, it's for a brief check-up. You've begun making the changes that we discussed last time, including tracking your habits and engaging in some aerobic exercise, as well as working on your mental focus and some novel learning experiences.

Now we're going to add another small change.

You've described a sense of craving toward some things in your life that you know aren't the healthiest, including sweet snacks and your favorite TV shows. So now we're going to experiment with a new strategy for dealing with those cravings.

- "When you feel the beginnings of a craving," I tell you, "your new prescription is to take a walk outside, to meditate, or to otherwise give yourself ten restful minutes before giving in to it."

As you leave my office, you're a bit surprised by this new prescription. Though you're skeptical about how this is really going to improve your health, you feel that waiting ten minutes isn't a huge deal. So you agree to give it a try.

EXTRA NOTE: TAKE-HOME THOUGHTS ABOUT SELF-CONTROL:

The following is a list of conditions or habits that deplete your energy and your self-control:

- mental illness
- chronic diseases
- sleep deprivation
- sedentary lifestyle
- processed foods and sugar
- tobacco
- alcohol and other drugs
- environmental exposures to toxins
- stressful environments (workplace and employers take note)

Compare this list to the following tally of habits that provide energy and *increase* self-control:

- having a healthy mind and body
- meditation

- practicing breath control

- exercise and movement

- getting adequate, restorative sleep

- plant-based, non-processed foods

- limiting exposures to toxins

- hydration

Take time to do a personal inventory of your own habits and state of health, and use these lists as a guide to consider what changes you can make today to gain energy and self-control that will help you move toward the future you desire.

ADDITIONAL RESOURCES

- *The Hacking of the American Mind: The Science Behind the Corporate Takeover of Our Bodies and Brains,* by Robert H. Lustig, M.D., MSL (I highly highly highly recommend this book)

- *The Willpower Instinct: How Self-Control Works, Why it Matters, and What You Can Do to Get More of it* by Kelly McGonigal, Ph.D.

- *Drug Dealer, MD: How Doctors Were Duped, Patients Got Hooked, and Why It's So Hard to Stop* by Anna Lembke, M.D.

- Simpleology, an app to establish new habit patterns

- HabitBull, a habit-tracking app available for iPhones and Androids

Unplugging: Intentional Stress Mastery with Breathing, Mindfulness, and Meditation

This chapter explains how uncontrolled stress responses are destructive to your health, then introduces practices that are powerful for reducing stress. You'll learn why mindfulness and meditation are necessary disciplines, and you'll find a simple process for developing a meditation practice. This method works, and it is foundational for everything else in this book.

THIS CHAPTER COULD strike you as a bit repetitive. That is intentional. I believe that chronic unmitigated stress is a major influencer of poor health. I believe this has only worsened in the information age. Our minds are continually assaulted by fear-provoking stimuli, and our bodies are staying in a perpetual low-grade fight-or- flight state of being. Fight-or-flight is great when we are truly threatened. However, this response becomes maladaptive when it is activated on a continual basis due to circumstances that really aren't threatening to us.

Mastering your stress requires an understanding that your brain is encountering stress whether you feel it or not. Chronic stress must be dealt with. You cannot hide from it. Fear is everywhere because fear sells. Fear makes money for somebody. Fear makes us behave in the way that those who sell fear want us to. We keep buying what they're selling. We watch their programs, eat addictive foods, consume addictive substances, or do whatever helps us feel better for just a moment. We hope someone will come up with a pharmaceutical or supplement that will make it a little easier.

These activities further deplete our energy and our ability to persevere courageously on our journey to being what we want to be. We are always becoming something. The question is, are you becoming what you want to be or are you becoming what others are conditioning you to be? It's your destiny, and you must take charge of it. In order to do so, you must master your own mind. That's why learning to meditate is a foundational habit for your health. In this time we live in, the skill of meditation is non negotiable. In quietude you will find your true self. In authentic rest you will find your strength.

Early in my medical career, I encountered a young professional who seemed, from the outside, to be doing very well. He had started his own business and had a family he loved. But when the economic crisis hit in 2008, his business struggled financially. He found himself feeling stressed and anxious about his circumstances. Typically an easy-going guy, he soon found that he frequently felt nervous and unsettled. He also began to wake at night and have trouble getting back to sleep. He found himself waking up already tired. Throughout his work week he would feel fatigued and sometimes short of breath. He had never had issues with anxiety or dealing with stress but this situation was different for him..

The story of what ultimately happened to him is the story of how intentional stress management can change everything—and how, without it, we're at the mercy of powerful negative forces.

This young professional had opened his business around the same time that he and his wife had started a family. They gave birth to three children in two years—twins first, then another. With this new family to support, he was lucky that his business grew quickly. His work was extremely demanding of his time and energy, and his life at home was, too. He found himself fatigued, but very happy.

His business was doing so well that he moved into a new, larger space. That was an exciting transition. But as soon as he'd gotten settled in a beautiful new office, the financial crisis hit. Suddenly the new space didn't seem so beautiful—just expensive. Pretty soon, his customers weren't coming through the door anymore, because they didn't have money in their pockets. He had only just finished paying off what he'd borrowed to get his business off the ground, and now he found himself having to borrow more money just to pay his bills. It seemed very possible that his entire business was going to fail and that his family's livelihood was hanging in the balance.

He did what anyone providing for three small children would have done: he worked harder. He showed up to the office earlier and worked later. He also did everything he could think of to build his business and bring in more customers.

Eventually, his efforts paid off. His business started to grow again. And as it did, he was able to start paying his bills again instead of borrowing. He also began, once again, to pay off his debts.

But the experience of nearly failing had taken a toll on him. He was now frequently feeling anxious and fearful that his business might still collapse. He found himself wondering if economic failure was just around the corner. He wondered how long it would take and how hard he would have to work to get himself and his family onto solid financial footing so he could finally relax. And every night, after a stressful day at his business and battling a continual feeling of unease, he went home to three small children who were hungry for his attention.

Before all of this happened, he had maintained healthy habits. He used to exercise and eat well. But he just didn't have time to exercise anymore. Sure, he was running around his office all day, but he didn't get outside for real physical activity. In fact, since a lot of this took place during the winter months, he would show up to his office in the dark and leave in the dark. He only saw the sun through the windows of his office.

He also had started to eat less. And frequently, he would realize that he hadn't once, during a twelve-hour workday, stopped to go to the bathroom. That meant he was dehydrated. He often felt weak and headachy, hungry and shaky.

This continued even after the financial problems had really subsided. His family was okay. His business was growing. Everything was going to be all right, yet he was continually chased by fear: what would happen if his business really did fail? How would he rebuild? How would he recover from all the debt?

The thing that finally made him change his direction might seem trivial. He was sitting exhausted and about to go to bed early one night when his wife turned on the movie *Eat, Pray, Love*. He didn't have any interest in it, but since he was too tired to get up, he couldn't help but watch a little.

Then he got drawn into the plot, and suddenly he found himself watching Julia Roberts meditate.

When the movie ended he was lying in bed, exhausted—and aware of his fear. He was aware of how he was still deeply afraid that a financial disaster was around the corner. He began to notice how far he was from the simplicity of "eat, pray, love."

"I'm tired of this," he thought. "I've got to find a way to get my energy back and find some peace. I've got to find a way to conquer fear."

He started to ask some simple questions. "Why am I so afraid?" he thought to himself.

And when he actually started to probe his anxiety, he realized he was spending all his time worrying about something that didn't deserve his worry at all.

His business had recovered. More than that, though, he suddenly saw that if his business really did fail, it wouldn't be the end of the world. He and his family would be okay. Yes, there would be a difficult period—but he would find a new job. He was confident in his ability to do that. Everything would be okay. And meanwhile, he had a wonderful spouse and three beautiful, healthy children.

Why had he allowed his life to become overrun by fear and anxiety?

Immediately, he began to seek out some valuable resources for stress management, which you'll find in the pages ahead. But the most important change had already taken place. He had seen his fears for what they were; he had seen that he could *choose* how to deal with them, rather than simply letting them control him. And he would never choose to let them control him again.

As it happens, that young professional was me. That was a very challenging period of my life. But because of it I learned—and personally tested—powerful techniques for mastering stress recommended by some of the most knowledgeable experts in the world. I can now share those techniques with you.

There will always be stress: for you, for me, for all of us. There is no making it go away. But each of us has a major choice to make in the way we choose to *manage* that stress. We can be intentional about what types of stress we expose ourselves to and what we do about stress once it's entered our psyche. It's extraordinarily powerful simply to recognize that we have that ability. In looking back at my own story, I know I did not need to be so afraid. I wish I could have understood that this was my path to further development and that I had the opportunity to embrace the situation as a chance for growth.

Let's break down what I was experiencing. I was going through a period of professional uncertainty due to circumstances that were beyond my control. This induced fear in me, because much of what I had worked for appeared to be vulnerable. But my overall fear was out of proportion to what I was actually facing. There really *was* uncertainty; circumstances were changing, and I couldn't do anything about that. But rather than identifying which circumstances were out of my control and which ones I could control, and then making a plan, I just simply started working harder and ignoring basic self-care principles.

Interestingly enough, working harder and being more proactive about trying to grow my business was exactly what I needed to do. But I didn't need to exhaust myself with a sense of fear each day. If I had been thinking clearly, I would have worked harder and been more proactive, but I also would have been realistic about the potential implications if things didn't work out. I didn't have to become exhausted by fear.

As it turns out, I'm now able to see that this was one of the most challenging and interesting times in my development, and that many of the great things that occurred down the road happened because of the stress of that moment. I learned many things about my business, my professional skills, and my family's supportive love of me. I also learned how much power my personal spiritual beliefs had to help me overcome fear. Now, in hindsight, I would not change those stressful circumstances. I embrace the idea that this period of time gave me a great opportunity to grow and thrive. And it was important for me to learn the lesson about fear and anxiety, and how exhausting it is, and to decide not to give it such power over me in the future.

The next time I go through a season like that—which I will—I hope that I'll be able to look at it through a positive lens rather than a negative one. I plan to maintain my healthy habits of breathing and sleeping and exercising and eating healthfully, and I plan to focus on enjoying whatever time I have away from the stressor, so that I don't hand over my emotional energy to circumstances that are beyond my control.

Most of all, this chapter is about awareness. It's about the type of awareness and mindfulness that we've talked about in the past two chapters. And it's about the same message that runs through everything in this book: that just about everything we do and just about everything we think is the result of habit. Thus *awareness* and *habit* are the context for everything that follows in this chapter and the rest of the book.

Awareness and habit are so important because, if we really look into the nature of things, we discover that we actually have very little control over the circumstances around us. Almost all the events of our lives are not under our direct control. But we do have control over how we interpret our circumstances and how we react to those circumstances, and over how we direct our energy toward the destinies that we envision for ourselves. *Those* are things over which we actually have power—and it is a profound, even life-changing power.

There are innumerable stories of people who have been in what we would consider intolerable circumstances, but who were able to create in their own minds a positive world that they could inhabit during that time. There are prisoners of war who spent years in isolation and yet, using their mental strength and their positive state of mind, were able to visualize themselves as moving toward a positive destiny.

In earlier chapters we talked about the difference between curing a disease versus simply treating, or palliating, the disease's symptoms. Most medications just palliate. Similarly, the vast majority of fads and gimmicks are meant to temporarily palliate a disease or merely distract from it; they don't attempt to cure the root problem.

So when we talk about stress mastery in this chapter we're seeking, as best we can, to address the root problem. We don't want merely to palliate the symptoms of stress.

And the cure is to look deeply into things. It's to be aware of what's impacting you, and to develop an emotional resiliency and courage. Our goal is to diminish the effects of fear, anxiety, and uncertainty on our state of being. It's to promote a mindset of courage, and from there to go into the positive emotions that provide energy—including joy, peace, and gratitude.

At the same time, it's important to note that some people suffer from significant psychological conditions. These are people who may have been born with a genetic disposition for a mental health disorder; in other cases, there are circumstances beyond anyone's control that may have impacted their ability to do the type of exercises, and experience the positive benefits, that this chapter is about.

Many of these individuals truly need medical care. I would encourage all of my readers who struggle with paralyzing fear, anxiety, panic disorders, or unstable moods that are impacting their relationships and their daily ability to function to consider a medical evaluation. If you have a severe mental health disorder, then seek care. Psychotherapy and medications may help you stabilize the condition and thereby give you a better chance at the healthy future you want. At the same time, the tools that you'll read about in this chapter will help just about everyone, including those with very severe mental health disorders.

For the vast majority of readers who primarily struggle with mild depression or negative thinking, the exercises in this chapter—when applied regularly—will be enough to change their mindset from a negative one to a positive one. That's our objective. We want to get you to a positive mindset, to where you're feeling courageous and in control of both your emotions and the way that you respond to the circumstances you can't control.

The tools that I'm going to outline below are powerful in this way. They sound simple; they might sound almost too easy to accomplish what I'm describing. But there are countless testimonies—from individuals over millennia of human existence—that give evidence to how effective these tools are.

I'm taking so much time to introduce this material because I want to emphasize how important it is. Your awareness of your emotional states and your stressors and your fears, as well as your recognition of what you can control and what you can't, is deeply important to your overall health. The cultivation of a positive mindset and the ability to enter into the present moment in a focused and effective and helpful way is also deeply important to your overall health.

I strongly encourage you to practice the techniques that you'll find in the following pages. First, I'm going to describe the physiological effects of stress, and then you'll find a few simple tools and some different ways of getting started. I have also posted many expanded resources on this topic at our web hub www.healthshepherds.com.

HOW STRESS AFFECTS YOU

Many of the people I see in my office are tired, depressed, physically sick, and taking numerous medications. But the root causes of their illnesses, in so many cases, are actually their own reactions to stress.

People come into my office with high blood pressure, reflux, irritable bowel syndrome, headaches, diffuse muscle pain, palpitations, shortness of breath, sleeplessness, depression, anxiety, fatigue, and many other conditions that often share a single underlying cause: fear.

When I'm in the exam room with a patient, I start out by asking about his or her physical illness. But when I'm facing someone who's anxious or stressed out, our conversation tends to reveal that there's something else going on: there are problems in the marriage, or in another key relationship, or in the family, or at work. And those problems are literally making them sick.

Sometimes the problems aren't in patients' immediate orbit, but they're devastated by what's going on in the world. They watch cable news every day and are worried sick about the imminent collapse of our government or about one tragedy after another in other parts of the world. And they're having very real health problems as a result of that nonstop mental stress.

The physiological effects of stress are real and profound. Stress raises blood pressure and can cause gastrointestinal symptoms. Stress causes our adrenal glands to secrete cortisol and catecholamines like adrenaline. It spikes blood sugar—and subsequently insulin—which increases the likelihood of obesity and diabetes. (This is the opposite of being lean and capable of burning fat effectively, as we talked about in Chapter Three.)

Stress also creates mental fatigue by consuming your cognitive functions. It creates unproductive brain activity that saps your energy and makes it difficult for you to concentrate on the things that actually require your attention. It affects your productivity and your ability to be in the present moment, whether the present moment includes family, friends, or professional responsibilities. As discussed earlier, stress depletes your self-control. It reduces your ability to choose in accordance with your highest desires.

When stress is sustained and uncontrolled over time, it can lead to physical pain, fatigue, acid reflux, irritable bowel, palpitations, perspiration, headaches, jaw tension, insomnia, and obesity, among other conditions. All of these are physical manifestations of stress. Stress also appears emotionally, as anxiety and depression or as anger, irritability, impatience, fear, negative or catastrophic thinking, or simply sadness. Many people experience a sense of helplessness that can be debilitating.

All of these conditions are deeply destructive to your mental and physical health. Luckily, they are largely preventable.

The prevention is to take control of your mind. The material in Chapter Four is foundationally important for this. You must know your own story and you must understand why you think, emote, and react the way you do. You have the ability to take control of your mind, then to take control of your responses to stress. You face a choice: either you will control your thinking—or others will control it for you.

THE FIRST STEP IS DETECTION; THE SECOND STEP IS INTERPRETATION

Whether your stress is manifesting in a physical or an emotional way, or both, it's important to be aware of what's happening. When a physical symptom or an unpleasant emotion arises, stop yourself and ask, "Where is this coming from?" The sooner you detect it, the better. You may very well be able to pinpoint precisely which situation or condition caused you to feel uncomfortable and then stressed.

So let's say you're in the midst of your workday and you notice that you're anxious and stressed out. The first thing to do is to acknowledge what you're feeling. That alone is something we often don't do, and the fact that we don't notice or acknowledge our emotions can lead to the feeling snowballing into irritability and then into a host of other feelings and conditions.

Next, think back to what's happened in your day. Sometimes it's easy to pinpoint the trigger and sometimes it isn't. (This will become easier with time, though, as you get accustomed to tuning into your stress responses.) But let's say you received an email about something important to you, and as you think back over your day, you recognize that was the trigger. You started to feel nervous or fearful when you read that email.

Now you've taken two important steps: you've acknowledged how you're feeling and you've identified its cause.

After detection comes interpretation. Because you've already accomplished the considerable feat of becoming aware of your stress and what's causing it, you now have a power that you didn't possess before: you can intentionally decide whether the situation is as significant as your stress response is making it out to be. You can reflect on whether this situation is actually important enough to allow your anxiety to harm your well-being in the way that it is.

Ask yourself a few questions. What exactly am I nervous about? What, precisely, am I afraid of? This allows your higher mind to do the work that it was designed to do, which is to read the many complicated signals you're receiving all at once and then to assess the situation.

Very often, the simple act of *identifying* the stress trigger is enough to defuse it. You'll discover that many stressors actually aren't worth as much emotional energy as you're devoting to them. Thus, just by detecting and naming it, you've done a lot of the work of dissolving it. You've noticed that this is something fairly minor in the larger scheme of things, and now it doesn't have the same power over you. It may no longer have enough power to make you stressed and unhappy.

This is why your *interpretation* of stressful events is hugely important. When I went through my own prolonged period of anxiety and stress, I was mostly wrong in my interpretation of what was happening in my life. I thought I was on the edge of economic ruin and that my entire life was about to come unraveled. In all that time, and in all that fear, I never stopped to think logically about what would actually happen if my business failed.

If that had really happened, I would have gotten a new job. I still had my medical degree and I could have gotten a job at a hospital or at another practice. I would have recovered. I was never actually facing doomsday. So I cannot stress enough—pun intended—that you've got to pay attention to the way you're interpreting the stress in your life. In one situation after another, you'll find that the circumstances don't really merit the extremity of your response.

At the same time, there *are* circumstances that are truly awful. People lose a loved one. People are diagnosed with cancer. Those situations warrant grief. For those who have gone through a genuinely traumatic event, I very much recommend working with a professional therapist. I am not at all suggesting that we should be emotionally neutral in every life event. But I am saying that we should apply the *right* emotional responses to the *right* situations in the *right* proportion—and that our health depends on it.

Sometimes a useful strategy is to think through a stressful situation to its worst possible outcome. So let's say that you know your company is going to have a round of layoffs in six months, and your anxiety over the possibility that you're going to lose your job is taking a huge toll on you.

You're stressed out; you're sleeping poorly at night. You're terrified that you're going to be among those who are laid off.

Instead of dwelling in that uncertainty, work through the situation in a logical way. Assume for a minute that you definitely *are* going to lose your job. So then you know that you've got six more months of a guaranteed paycheck ahead of you, or perhaps a bit more if your employer offers some severance. Suddenly, with the layoff becoming a certainty instead of a hypothetical, it's clear that worrying about it won't do you any good. All you can do now is take control of the situation.

Then start to think methodically about how you're going to respond. You consider the market opportunities for yourself. You draw up a plan for your family: How are we going to get through this time? Maybe you remember that a friend or a family member dealt with a layoff and a period of unemployment. How did they deal with it?

You realize that it didn't devastate their family; they're doing just fine now. But there was a period of adjustment. They made some changes during that time. Maybe they had to relocate for a new job. But everything worked out in the end. Sometimes things actually work out even better than they were before; sometimes a layoff turns out to be a blessing in disguise.

So now you've got a plan. You've freshened up your résumé and identified job opportunities for yourself. You know which changes you and your family will have to make to tighten your belts during a spell of unemployment. And though you still feel unhappy at the prospect of losing your job, you see that you'll be okay. You've made your plan. And because of it, maybe you even find that you can move forward with confidence.

Sometimes, our stressors aren't personal. We often fail to realize that the cumulative exposure to the twenty-four-hour news cycle—and to social media, email, and the Internet generally—are all elevating our stress levels. Think about it from a biological perspective. The human mind wasn't intended, before even fully waking in the morning, to be exposed to information about how thousands of people on the other side of the world died in a mudslide. For almost all of human history we wouldn't even have known that happened. Now we try to get our minds around these catastrophes the instant we check our devices in the morning or turn on the news or radio. We feel awful about them; we wonder what it would be like if that had happened to us. And as we do so, all of our stress responses are through the roof.

On top of that, many of the news stations and websites that we tune into on a daily basis are intentionally and artificially elevating our fear responses—because sensationalism sells. They want us to stay with them longer and to come back again and again. But you're going to have to decide: will you allow yourself to be manipulated by media outlets that are just trying to make money? Or will you take charge of your own emotions?

This chapter would not be complete if we did not at least mention the direct negative impact that our devices are having on our brains. It is not just the information overload from the devices causing the problem. It is the cumulative exposure to the light frequencies, electromagnetic energy, and the loss of awareness when we are focused on our phone, tablet, or computer for so much of our day. Our minds are designed to engage in the real world with real people. This is especially true for our children. There is emerging evidence that our smartphones are directly contributing to ADD, depression, anxiety, insomnia, and other psychological conditions for both us and our children. We have to place some boundaries on our use of screens, especially for our children. This topic is explored more deeply on my web hub. For now, just know it is really important to limit your exposure.

THE POWER OF CONTROLLING YOUR BREATH

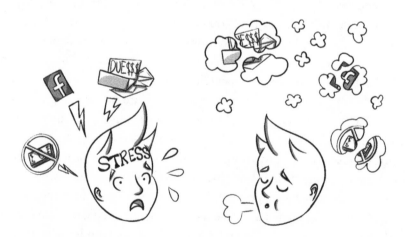

As with everything you've read so far in this book, responding in a healthy way to the stressful conditions of your life comes through developing positive habits. In the coming pages, you'll find a medicine for tackling stress that doesn't require a prescription and is entirely free. It will also start to deliver benefits as soon as you begin using it. Actually, just a couple minutes of practice will be enough for you to feel a little better.

The real key, though, is to take steps to manage your stress regularly. In order to truly improve your health, intentional stress management has to become a habit. Once it's a habit, you won't have trouble maintaining it.

Some of the Eastern meditation traditions call the habit of negative and distracted thinking "monkey brain." And if you think about it, that's a really good name for it. Consider all the emotions bouncing around in your mind: all the negative interpretations, the worries about things that will never actually happen, the way you're distracted from one thing to the next to the next. It really *is* like a bunch of monkeys jumping around in your brain. It's accomplishing nothing.

The stress management techniques that I'm about to share with you have the goal of turning off monkey brain and turning on your deeper, more intuitive brain. This deeper part of your brain—which is called the "witness" in Eastern tradition—has the ability to guide your thoughts and give you the right kind of focus. It's the part of your brain that's capable of evaluating your own thinking and your own emotions to decide which interpretations make sense and which are unhelpful and should be turned off.

Most of us are so stuck in "monkey brain" mode that we're not even aware that we have a "witness" inside of us. But we do. *You* do. In witness mode, you'll notice a negative emotion as you experience it, and you'll look to its root cause. Sometimes that will mean looking at your least-becoming qualities, such as anger or jealousy. But the witness sees these qualities to their root and then helps us to deal with them authentically. Eventually, our negative emotions—jealousy and spite, shame and despair—can become their positive correlates, like courage, commitment, and acceptance. The witness is a route to a deeper peace that most of us experience only rarely.

The means of cultivating this higher mind begins in something very simple: controlled breathing (there are many forms of breathwork referred to by various names). That might sound strange, but in fact, this is a powerful and effective strategy for productively directing your concentration. It's also non-negotiable if you're after genuine good health. Controlled breathing is a practice that will take a little while to develop and will require some patience, but the end result is extraordinary: emotional resiliency. It's the ability to step into life with courage and then to maintain a state of relative peace in the face of tremendous stress.

You now know that I've struggled with all of this myself. When I first realized that I needed to calm myself down, I tried to focus on my breathing because of the many studies demonstrating how breathwork exercises can reduce stress responses. But at first it didn't work. I tried sitting down to practice first thing in the morning. I would get into a comfortable position, and then I'd start breathing deeply and counting my breaths. But within seconds, my brain would say, "What are you doing? You've got a million things to do this morning. This is a waste of time. Get up and start doing something."

So I stopped.

But I was so determined to conquer fear that pretty soon I tried it again. The same thing happened. I stopped again. And then I tried it again. Eventually, I was able to really stick with it—because I was absolutely determined to find a way to quiet my mind and experience real peace, and it seemed that controlled breathing and meditation were necessary for this to happen. And finally, it worked.

As I was trying to develop this practice, I was also aware that I would sometimes experience spontaneous shortness of breath and that practicing breathwork was the way to resolve that issue. Interestingly enough, I became really aware of my own shortness of breath by frequently seeing patients who had the same problem. Patients came to see me all the time who said they were afraid they had lung disease or heart disease or some other problem because they often found themselves out of breath and needing to stop simply to breathe.

When I inquired about their symptoms, though, I usually determined that the problem was simply due to ineffective breathing. I always did the appropriate medical evaluations, of course—checking vital signs, oxygen level, making sure they weren't anemic, and so on—but the results almost always showed normal functioning. Their shortness of breath was a reflection of dysfunctional breathing habits. This could be due to over-breathing or under-breathing.

All day long, they were taking short and shallow breaths with their mouth and chest. They were not using their respiratory system as it was designed which is to breathe through the nose and use the diaphragm. I was doing something similar. I was running from one patient to the next all day, and when I'd sit down with a patient, I paid no attention to my posture. I wasn't hydrating. And I certainly wasn't taking the time to pay attention to my breathing. Meanwhile, my brain was sensing this and, as a result, periodically sent me messages to stop and take some breaths. That's all it was.

When I described this to my patients, they almost always said, "Yeah, you know, that makes sense." Very often, these patients were carrying around an extra twenty pounds and weren't paying attention to their posture. They tended to slump forward, which meant that their chest wasn't thoroughly expanding. Then they would sit at a desk all day and that belly would push up against their diaphragm, restricting their breathing.

We tend not to think about it, but our breathing machinery—that is, our "pulmonary" system—performs a vital function and needs to be intentionally exercised. Yet most of us don't do that, and then we find our breathing has become restricted. I have created a resource with a more thorough description of this function with examples of different forms of breathing exercises on our web hub.

The average person who comes into my office takes probably fifteen breaths a minute, or one every four seconds, and uses approximately a third of their lung capacity. That's what I was doing, too, before I tried the controlled breathing practice. But using just a third of your lung capacity isn't good for your health.

You're now going to start training yourself to engage in a deeper type of breathing that will make you feel physically healthier. And as you do it, you'll develop a powerful resilience to the many stressors of daily life.

I also want to emphasize that this habit of breath control is as important to your health as drinking water, eating food, and sleeping. Our minds are so over-stimulated that they are literally starved for restorative periods of quiet. In my earlier years, there were ample quiet spaces for reflection. We now live in a time where information and stimulation are crammed into every moment and we are constantly deprived of quiet, reflective time. If you do not honor your brain's need for reflection, meditation, and periods of stillness, you will break down, both physically and mentally.

The next several pages introduce techniques for controlled breathing that will help you to breathe deeply to support your mental and physical health. Note that controlled breathing is not the same as meditation, though they are related. Controlled breathing teaches you how to deepen and focus your breathing to reduce acute stress, improve your energy, and improve your mental fortitude. Meditation is diverse with many different approaches and purposes. For the purposes of this book, meditation will be the use of a focusing vehicle to induce your brain into a deeply restful, restorative, and calm state. This will help you diffuse the effects of chronic stress on your mind, body, and emotions.

Scientifically speaking, meditation is a powerful brain training exercise. Meditation increases blood flow to your prefrontal cortex, that powerful thinking center in your brain. Meditation reduces activity in your flight-or-fight systems. Meditation increases willpower. As you practice different types of meditation and breath control, you begin to condition your brain to occupy a calm and focused state in response to how you are breathing. You can use your breath to regain control of your brain.

Let me take a moment to emphasize that I am not a meditation teacher. I am a meditator and have studied various forms of meditation for years, but I am not an instructor. My goal is to get you started. I would encourage you to take a meditation course or use one of the resources listed at the end of this chapter to deepen your practice. My personal meditation is about thirty minutes daily split between morning and afternoon sessions. It does not take much time, and what it gives back to me is far greater than the little bit of time I give up to practice this skill. I started years ago with just five minutes daily. Meditation is free, requires no special gear or equipment, and requires minimal physical effort.

However, meditation requires mental effort. We are giving you a tool to build your brain. Building new connections in your brain and strengthening the communication between your right and left brain requires energy. Even though meditation is rest, it will feel like effort. All things worth having require effort. Your brain is a thinking organ. Your brain thinks; that's what it does. You cannot stop your brain from thinking any more than you can stop your heart from beating. When you start to practice these techniques, expect to continue to experience your thoughts. Not being able to shut off your brain is not an excuse to not meditate. It is the reason you need to meditate. Your conditioned thinking patterns and emotional responses will resist your efforts to develop new thinking pathways. Do not judge yourself for this resistance or become frustrated by it. Instead, expect resistance and do not be surprised by it. Just remind yourself of what you're trying to achieve and continue your meditation.

The breathing practices that you are about to learn have been taught as an essential discipline for thousands of years, across all faiths and existential worldviews. This is for everyone. It can be integrated into any faith system or set of beliefs. Over the years, I personally have integrated this practice into my own faith observance, and vice versa—to powerful effect.

EFFECTIVE BREATHING IN THREE PHASES

To begin this practice, it's important for you to know that your posture is paramount to your breathing. You need to get your body into a good, neutrally aligned position to breathe effectively. Many of us hold our bodies in ways that are so restrictive that when we attempt to breathe deeply, we actually end up putting *more* stress on our bodies instead of less. As you breathe, note that your ribcage should move *outward* more than upward. Again, refer to the image provided.

To help you better visualize this process we've created a short video to demonstrate proper breathing, available through www.healthshepherds. com.

I will now describe this effective breathing in phases.

◆ Phase One

Start out simply by focusing your attention on your breathing and by inhaling through your nose. Take deep breaths so that it feels like you're filling up your belly. (You're not really breathing into your belly, of course; that's just what it feels like.) It's important not to increase your abdominal pressure while doing this; that is, you should feel your belly gently rise, but you shouldn't feel *pressure* in your belly. Refer again to the image provided so that you're maintaining the correct posture. Indeed, try not to put *pressure* on yourself to breathe. This is meant to be a lifelong practice; we don't want to pressure ourselves. Instead, we want to slowly improve our ability to breathe well and to be patient with our bodies as we adapt to this.

As you exhale, it should feel like you're emptying your belly. Your navel should pull back toward your spine as you exhale. As you do this, simply keep your attention on your breath, noticing how your belly expands and contracts.

◆ Phase Two

In the second phase, you're going to actually use your ribcage and your respiratory muscles that surround your chest wall. These muscles are probably deconditioned, in the same way our muscles generally get out of shape when we don't exercise them. For this reason, in this second phase, it's perfectly normal to become short of breath.

In the first phase, you focused on the feeling of your belly expanding and contracting. Now turn that focus to your chest and ribcage. Take a deep breath through your nose in the same way that you did before, but now allow your ribcage and chest to expand and rise. You should feel your chest pulling outward more than upward. Then exhale, noticing how your chest and ribcage contract.

You're now using muscles that don't get a lot of use and you've begun to transform your breathing from the short, shallow breaths that most people use into a deeper, healthier, and more controlled form of breathing that exercises your pulmonary system.

◆ Phase Three

In the final phase of effective breathing, you start out breathing in the same way that you did in the second phase. But now, during your inhale, after your ribcage is already full of air, you're going to pull air into your upper lungs and chest. This will be the hardest part. You'll feel the air coming into the collarbone area. You'll probably feel a tight pull in your chest, or a wheeze. That's completely normal. You should keep pulling air into this area until you feel you cannot do it any longer. And yet, as you reach your capacity, you should be able to stop calmly—that is, you should not feel like you're gasping or putting a lot of pressure on your chest.

Exhale exactly the same way: empty the upper chest, feel your ribcage and chest wall contract, and notice as your navel pulls down to your belly. You're now fully inhaling and fully exhaling. With practice, you'll begin to combine the three phases into an integrated sequence that eventually will become one smooth motion.

Whereas most people breathe about fifteen times per minute and use a fraction of their lung capacity, this technique gets you to spend eight or nine seconds on a single breath and to use much more of your lung capacity in doing so. Once you've gotten somewhat comfortable with this practice, set a goal for yourself to inhale for seven or eight seconds and to exhale for twice as many seconds as you breathed in. Experiment with pausing in between breaths. Eventually, you'll be able to take just four or five breaths (or less) per minute instead of fifteen. With regular practice, you may even find that you can take *thirty*-second smooth easy breaths.

When you first try this deep breathing, I can pretty much promise that you'll feel like you're not good at it. You'll probably have to catch your breath from all the breathing—which seems strange. It will seem like something's wrong. But nothing's wrong. You're just training your body into a new habit.

That's why you should practice this type of breathing as much as you can. It's going to condition you in the same way that exercise does. You're going to feel better in your body and your brain. And when you feel stressed and short of breath, you'll suddenly have a powerful tool available to you. It may not seem powerful right now, but it will.

This technique will also eventually allow you to put yourself to sleep at night. It won't work for that right away, because at first it's challenging and will make you more alert. But later on, you'll be able to use this breathing to get into a meditative state and to turn off that monkey brain.

◆ Box breathing

Another important controlled breathing technique is called "box" breathing. A Navy SEAL, Mark Divine, gave it that name in his book *Unbeatable Mind*; he calls it box breathing because it has four equal parts. I've found this type of breathing to be particularly effective for enhancing focus.

In the first step, you take the kind of deep inhale—into your upper chest—that you learned in the description of effective breathing above. You breathe into your belly, you expand your chest, and then you pull air into your upper chest. In the second step of box breathing, you calmly stop inhaling and simply hold that air in. Then, in the third step, you exhale. Finally, in the fourth step, you once again stop and pause before taking a new inhale. The essential part of all this is that you do each of these four steps for an equal amount of time.

To do that, you first determine what you're capable of. Maybe you can inhale for a maximum of four seconds. In that case you inhale for four seconds, hold it for four seconds, exhale for four seconds, and hold that for another four seconds. The entire four-part sequence takes sixteen seconds, and then you start again. Count your breaths as you do it. That's an important part of the process, because it forces you to focus your mind.

At first, as with the previous type of breathing, you'll probably have to stop and catch your breath after box breathing. But eventually, your body will develop the capacity. I started out only being able to inhale for a few seconds, but after practicing for a while I got to the point where I could inhale for ten seconds. That meant I could do one cycle of box breathing for forty seconds. I was also able to sustain that rate for fifteen minutes or more if desired. It was an enormous improvement relative to where I'd started.

As I improved, I continued to count my breaths as I had at the start of the practice. After a while, though, I found that I didn't necessarily need to count anymore. I found myself naturally turning off my monkey brain and turning on my witness. I was able to think creatively and purposefully about the day ahead of me, and what I wanted to accomplish. I could do some positive thinking around my purpose and goals, both professionally and personally.

That morning breathing session became a very productive routine for me. I got to the point where you couldn't keep me from it. I did my fifteen minutes of box breathing each morning and I applied some positive visualization, and I got so that I was genuinely excited about each day ahead of me.

Of course, I still experienced stress throughout the day. I continued to run into problems and the general dysfunction of life, and sometimes I would find myself growing irritable or impatient or short of breath, just as I had before. But now I knew to stop myself. I got into the habit of stopping and asking, "Why is this happening?" I'd step into a quiet place for two minutes of box breathing. And when I did that, I was able to see that the problem I was facing was minor in the scheme of my life. I was able to refocus on what I wanted to accomplish and then return to my day.

Over time, becoming practiced in controlled breathing delivers a host of health benefits. You'll build the kind of learning synapses in your brain that allow you to focus more effectively instead of always becoming distracted or spiraling into a negative thinking loop. You'll improve your cognitive function.

And during stressful situations, you'll be calmer than you were before—which means you'll be more likely to find a productive solution to something stressful. In other words, you'll have more courage and more confidence, and you'll be a better problem solver.

You'll also become more emotionally intelligent. You'll begin to recognize your own emotions and enter into them as intentionally as possible. You'll see the root causes of your negative feelings and, through that, you'll know yourself better. That will help you to have more grace in the way that you move through your life. You'll be less inclined to judge others harshly, which will make you a source of positivity for those around you.

MEDITATION FOR YOUR HEALTH

Focused breathing is a great relaxation tool and strengthens the mind. The practice of meditation is a little different. As stated earlier, there are many forms of meditation. We have been emphasizing throughout this book the concept of mindfulness. Mindfulness meditation will bring you into the present moment and reduce acute stress responses. There are many different tools for mindfulness meditation, and I list a few at the end of the chapter.

With this type of meditation, we use our breath as a focusing vehicle that initiates the desired response in our mind. We focus on breath awareness, but do not put a lot of effort into our actual breathing. We just want to be aware of our breath and use it to calm our thinking and relax our bodies. I am going to provide you with a basic formula for how to do this, but it's beyond the scope of this book to teach this in a detailed manner. There are many guided meditation resources available to help you cultivate this skill.

I want you to start by finding a quiet and comfortable place. It's best if you find a time where you will not be disturbed or interrupted during your meditation. However, as you develop the skill, you will find yourself able to meditate in almost any environment no matter how distracting. This is one of the benefits of meditating. You can simultaneously manage your responsibilities while staying more connected to your higher mind. Set a timer without an alarm for the amount of time you would like to meditate. We want to finish our meditation quietly and not have a stressful alarm pull us out of our relaxed state abruptly. It's okay to glance at the timer occasionally if needed.

I would suggest you sit in a comfortable position with your back supported but your head and neck free. I do not suggest lying down as you may go to sleep, which while great for getting rest, is not the primary point of meditation. If you prefer to sit without your back supported or with your legs crossed, that is fine. However, I want you to be physically comfortable to best enable entering a deeply restful state during your meditation.

Once you're comfortable, close your eyes and begin to notice your breath. You may feel your breath in your nose, neck, chest, abdomen, or all of the above. Just notice how your breath feels to you. You may choose to count your breaths. You may count each breath, count the duration of the inhale and the exhale, or quietly count throughout the breath. You just want to focus on your breath. You will certainly find that your thoughts began to distract you from your breath. That is normal. Once you realize you have become distracted, just return to your breath. Every time you find yourself thinking, worrying, or problem-solving, just return to your breath for whatever time you have set aside for this purpose.

At the end of this time, take a minute or two to focus on what you are grateful for. Finishing your meditation with a gratitude exercise will increase the benefits of your meditation. You could start with just five minutes and gradually increase your time as you desire. You can use short versions of this process to reduce stress throughout your day. Try to practice this every day.

It's normal to find this process challenging. If you do this for five minutes, you may literally feel that you spent four minutes and fifty seconds with your mind racing. However, it will not be long until you find yourself in a calm and relaxed state for four minutes out of five. Some meditations will feel deeply effective; others not so much. Try not to judge one versus the other. You are on a long-term journey for the health of your mind. Every meditation, no matter how it felt, will do something good for you.

Mindfulness meditation is a great starting place. There are forms of meditation that use different focusing vehicles to provide a very deep level of rest for the brain and body. These are very effective for reversing the negative effects of chronic stress. I personally use one of these types of meditations as my primary meditation. I use breath control techniques and mindfulness practices throughout my day for different purposes. However, I use a mantra-based practice for my steady diet of meditation for my mental and physical health. I integrate this with spiritual practices associated with my personal faith. In the chapter resources I provide information for an organization that instructs people on this type of meditation. I encourage you to explore this option. Although similar, mindfulness and meditation are actually two distinct practices. It is important to learn both. I created a document describing the differences that is available on our web hub.

A WEALTH OF RESOURCES FOR CULTIVATING A PURPOSEFUL PRESENT

This chapter has only scratched the surface of the powerful breathing and meditative techniques that are available to you for managing the stress of daily life. I've intentionally presented only a couple of techniques in order to keep things simple. But that doesn't mean you should stop here. I'm including a list of additional materials for those who would like to go further.

If you find that you generally see things from a negative point of view, or if you tend to hold on to negative emotions such as anger, bitterness, or a lack of forgiveness—or if you find that the circumstances of your life have left you with an overall negative disposition—I would especially recommend that you look at my list of resources and explore additional materials. There is evidence to indicate that many of these exercises are actually more effective for curing mild to moderate depression and anxiety disorders than psychotherapy or medication. You can actually *cure* these conditions with these exercises!

In particular, I would point to the book Flourish by psychologist Martin Seligman, as well as his associated online resources at www.authentichappiness.sas.upenn.edu . On this website, you'll find free measurement tools to assess your strengths and your particular mindset. You'll also find exercises that, when practiced regularly, have proven effective for overcoming negative thinking and developing positive thinking. I strongly encourage you to use these source materials.

If, on the other hand, you're someone who has a mostly positive rather than negative mindset, and if you already find yourself feeling grateful most of the time, the specific techniques I described above will still be useful. They will help you become more relaxed and better enjoy the present moment, as well as become more focused and improve your performance at the right times. They are also some of the most powerful tools for in-ducing sleep, once they've become a regular habit.

These tools can also be integrated into any other form of contem-plative meditation. Meditation has many purposes; it can be used to pro-vide positive visualization, enhance creativity, or to form plans for your personal or professional life. It can be used to help you focus in a given moment and apply your best resources to the task at hand. It can be used to reduce anxiety or stress responses so you can physically and emotionally calm down when you're feeling overwhelmed. It can be used to enhance your ability to get to sleep, either in the evening or if you wake during the night. It can be integrated with a perspective of gratitude or appreciation of beauty, or with your particular faith.

Similarly, meditation can be used to enhance your enjoyment of the outdoors and activities such as hiking. It can be integrated into something as simple as relaxing in a park or sitting at a city cafe and watching the peo-ple go by. The better you get at it, the more you'll be able to diversify how you use meditation to get into a focused state, even while remaining alert in your environment. That, in turn, will improve your habits of thinking, your emotional awareness, and your strength of mind.

These tools are powerful no matter how you practice them—even if you only do a couple of minutes here and there. But remember, the pur-pose of this work isn't to do only a few minutes once in a while. The pur-pose is to usher a deeper focus into your daily life.

Studies have also shown that more frequent, shorter periods of these exercises are more effective than longer, infrequent sessions. In other words, five minutes every day is better than forty-five minutes once a week.

"Live in the present" is a cliché, of course. But hardly anyone actually does it. It's difficult to really live in the present. We have so many responsi-bilities, and we're constantly trying to get everything done while also plan-ning what's next. At the same time, our devices are continually distracting us into their digital world. Remember that focused breathing and medita-tion is your doorway into the present. It's your route to taking control of this moment—and to making it purposeful.

STEP INTO THE CONSULTATION ROOM

When you come in for your next exam, you mention that you tend to worry a lot, and we circle back to your family history and the fact that one of your parents suffers from depression. We discuss the possibility of a prescription for an antidepressant—but it's not entirely clear that you need medication. You worry about your kids, about money, and about whether there are going to be layoffs at your job if the economy doesn't improve. You also find yourself frequently disturbed by the stuff you hear on the news, like mass shootings. Your mood is often low, and you don't feel as much motivation as you'd like. Once again, we decide to focus on your habits.

Your new health program already contains the following:

- Daily journaling about your habit, which includes identifying which habits are moving you toward health and which are doing the opposite.
- Exercises designed to strengthen your mind and thinking, including engaging in novel learning experiences.
- When you feel the beginnings of a craving, you go for a walk, meditate, or otherwise give yourself ten restful minutes before giving in to the craving.

Now we add one more:

- Five minutes of deep breathing and focus exercises each morning and evening.

After agreeing to this new plan, we decide that you'll check in with me in a few weeks. You're not at all sure that breathing exercises will be enough to solve your problems—but you leave the appointment feeling hopeful.

FURTHER READING, LISTENING, AND OTHER EXPLORATION:
- *Unbeatable Mind* by Mark Divine
- *Anatomy of the Soul* by Curt Thompson, M.D. (Christian)
- *The Pema Chodron Audio Collection* (Audiobook; Zen Buddhist)
- Oak Meditation oakmeditation.com, An outstanding guided

breathing and meditation app.

- Ziva Online zivameditation.com, An excellent 8 day online meditation course that teaches a mantra based meditation. I highly recommend this course. If you choose to explore this option, stop by www.healthshepherds.com and click on the meditation tab. Ziva Online has offered a discount code for those who sign up. I have no financial relationship with Ziva meditation. I just like their course.

- Breathwork- Wim Hof Method. *The Oxygen Advantage,* by Patrick Mckeown

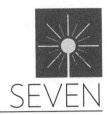

SEVEN

Nutrition: Cutting Through the Confusion

This chapter provides a sustainable approach to eating in a manner that supports healthy weight and energy. By learning how to source your food properly and how to become mindful about your eating habits, you'll overcome dysfunctional eating and promote lifelong health. You will learn how to provide your body with the nutrients necessary to experience your best health.

THE GOAL OF this chapter is to inspire you to have a healthy mindset about food. Our mindset about food has become dysfunctional. We have an overabundance of cheap, low-quality, and often habit-forming foods that we eat at a frequency inconsistent with our actual needs. We eat for the wrong reasons and often choose foods that are potentially more harmful than helpful. These choices start very early in our lives. As children, we have cartoon characters beckoning us to enjoy cereals with high-fructose corn syrup, artificial dyes, and preservatives. We become habituated sugar eaters before we even know what food is or what it is for.

Our medical recommendations, while well intentioned, often have not helped the situation. We took natural butter off our tables and replaced it with synthetic margarines because they were supposedly healthier. Now those same synthetic fats carry warning labels on them. We rightly vilified Joe Camel for influencing our youth to try nicotine, but we did not notice the myriad of cartoon characters influencing our children to eat sugar (a likely addictive substance). It is time to restore our mindset about food and our approach to eating.. This is an absolute necessity if you want authentic health for yourself and your children.

Food is far more than fuel. Food is sustenance. Food does contain fuel, but it also contains so much more. When we reduce food to just being fuel, we reduce our bodies to just being machines. Our bodies are far more than machines. Our bodies are infinitely complex systems. We need sustenance and experience authentic pleasure when we consume nutritious foods. We experience false pleasure when we consume sugary, heavily processed foods. This experience leads to the craving pathway we discussed earlier. We want our food to provide authentic and sustained well-being. We must restore our relationship to food.

Take a few minutes to consider these questions:

- What is food for you?
- Are you controlled by food or do you choose your food?
- What would you like food to be for you?
- What do you imagine it could be for you?

This chapter will help you restore your relationship to food and let it be for you what it should be: energy, health, life, pleasure, balance. We start by getting rid of all the poor-quality foods and helping your body and mind recover from your prior dysfunctional eating habits. We then slowly add back healthy foods over time and help you discover how tasty and pleasing nutritious foods can be. We then set you free to individualize your long-term nutrition plan in a manner that vitalizes your relationship to food and supports your best health. You will never regret restoring your relationship to food.

I want to make it clear that I enjoy food and believe we should all enjoy food. I am emphatic in my messaging about nutrition because of the current epidemic of diseases that are strongly influenced by our current approach to eating. When it is time to eat, I eat. I enjoy feasting with my friends and family. I do not think we should be obsessing about food. We just need to approach it from the right perspective.

There are probably three relatively broad groups of people who may end up reading this book. The first is a person who is pretty healthy and feels good most of the time. Perhaps they were just curious about the content. They do not really need to change much about their habits, but maybe they could improve their nutrition and stress management a little. Maybe they find this information helpful.

The second are people who are currently overweight or obese, and who already have the warning signs of chronic diseases. They may have been told that they have pre-diabetes, borderline hypertension, or high triglycerides. They may lack energy, or they may think they feel just fine. They do not have to change yet, but if they do not, they will become sick. This group, if they can follow the general principles of this book, can reverse these developing diseases and improve how they feel. I would wager that even those who think they feel fine would realize a significant improvement in daily energy if they made the changes I am recommending. It is important for these people to really use the power of their minds to catalyze the changes they need to make.

The third group is obese and sick. They have been diagnosed with diseases and take medications to control them. They more than likely feel bad most of the time. Their poor health is seriously impacting their quality of life and their ability to function well. This group needs to change. If they do not, they will become much sicker. This group really needs to examine their nutrition. They need to understand how to adopt an approach to eating that can help them begin to restore their health.

Depending on which group you are in, you may find you can be more permissive in your approach to eating. If you are in the third group, you probably need to take this content very seriously and try to apply it 90-100% of the time if you can. If you are in the second group, you can probably apply these principles 80% of the time and still gradually reach your goals for your health. By monitoring how you feel, your weight, and your biometrics, you will know if what you are doing is working.

This book is a starting place. Once you are back in control of your eating habits, you will want to dive deep into the resources that can help you prepare nutritious and tasty meals. This book is not a recipe book. There are already many great recipe books available for you to explore.

One final note. I am currently working toward a certificate in nutritional coaching and behavioral change methodologies through Precision Nutrition, an evidence-based nutritional coaching organization. This book just scratches the surface of nutrition. Nutrition is an amazingly complex topic, and research is always forthcoming to help us better understand nutrition. Our web resource hub www.healthshepherds.com will be a source for continual education about nutrition.

This chapter is meant to simplify things and give people a basic formula for healthy nutrition that works for them. I believe the vast majority of people can achieve an ideal body weight and support their good health by just following the advice in this chapter. However, if you want to understand the details of the ketogenic diet, or the lower inflammation diet, or the reset-your-gut microbiome diet, you will need more information than this chapter provides. Our web hub can help you find the answers to those questions. Most of you do not want to have to think that much about it. This chapter, while lengthy, should give you most of what you need to know. Take your time with this chapter. Do not be in a hurry. The victory of forming a healthy approach to eating happens in the mind. Once you have won the battle in your mind, the rest becomes easy.

This chapter describes a comprehensive approach to eating. However, if you would like access to the 9-week structured program to initiate weight loss that we designed, it is available for download or viewing at www.healthshepherds.com. If you would like a structured eating plan to initiate weight loss, gain control of your hunger, and improve your food sourcing, our program will help. It is not necessary to use our 9-week curriculum. You can apply the general principles of this chapter and gradually improve your metabolism and your health. You may prefer to adopt a fasting routine to help with weight loss. However, if you want a structured plan, the 9-week program is available on our web hub along with other resources about nutrition.

I want to make it very clear that sustained calorie restricted diets do not provide long-term weight loss. If you overeat, then eating less will be necessary to lose weight. However, we do not want to undereat in a sustained manner. All you really need to do is allow your eating habits and the foods you eat to provide your body with the information it needs to give you back your best health. The main themes of this chapter are to be mindful about eating, choose truly nutritious foods, eliminate foods that make you sick, and balance feeding and fasting. That's it. The rest of this chapter explains these principles.

I do include sample eating programs as a starting place. However, I am not a fan of non-individualized diets. Your genetics, your gut micro-biome, your circadian rhythms, your geographical location, your ancestry, and many other factors all influence your best diet. My food tables are not comprehensive. They are a starting place. I encourage you to review the additional teachings on our web hub for a more comprehensive under-standing of nutrition. I also present case studies of actual patients who have changed their nutrition and changed their health. Their stories may help you on your quest for your best health.

You're now savvy to the fact that the nutrients in the foods you eat be-come the energy that fuels you in body and mind. And while it's probably obvious that you can't survive without nutrients, it might be less obvious that your body requires certain kinds of nutrients in order to function properly. If your body isn't getting the right nutrients from the right sourc-es, you'll feel drained of energy, and that will affect the way you engage with your life each day. It will affect your ability to do your job, to think clearly, to enjoy your time with family and friends, and to pursue your pur-pose in life, whatever your unique purpose may be.

Unfortunately, millions of Americans currently find themselves in that very situation. This chapter contains the information about nutrition that I started providing to our patients to help them find their way back to good health.

This approach isn't focused on weight loss, though you'll very likely lose weight as a result of it—and you may lose a great deal of weight. This approach is about addressing a crisis; so many people suffer from poor nu-trition, but the resources to genuinely improve their health and treat their obesity are out of reach. The help they need is too expensive, or it's not covered by insurance, or it's too difficult for patients to maintain certain programs on a consistent basis. It's clear that many people aren't getting the help they need.

The nutritional approach that you'll find here has been hugely suc-cessful for patients dealing with a wide variety of health problems, from a lack of energy and chronic physical pain to morbid obesity. The program is designed to help you recreate the proper physiological processes that you read about in Chapter Three, so that your body stores and uses energy as it's supposed to. And it's intended to be sustainable for the long term, unlike many of the fad and crash diets that are popular today.

This approach has allowed patients to reverse their diseases. It's allowed people to lose a lot of weight. It has allowed people with insulin-dependent type 2 diabetes to come off their insulin. It has allowed people to stop taking their blood pressure medications and their reflux medications, and to stop using their CPAP machines. People who began to adopt nutritional changes as part of their medical treatment plan became healthier and felt profoundly better. They stopped giving away their energy to sickness and begin to apply their energy to their purpose.

They achieved all of that by making this approach their habit. You now understand that everything is a habit. How you eat is certainly a habit. Whether you snack or not, and how much you snack, are habits. You might be conscious of your habits, or you might not be, but they're still very much habits. And they're probably habits that you acquired over a long period of time as a result of the culture and the people around you.

To make this approach work for you, and in order to make it your habit, you have to *desire* it. No one can want it for you; you're the only one with the power to change your habits. So take a second to reflect on the goals you hold for your own health. Visualize the healthy version of yourself that you're striving for. This isn't about making a change to achieve short-term results; this is about desiring your good health so passionately that you're in it for the long haul.

You're going to need every ounce of that desire, because, unfortunately, our food industry isn't going to help you make this new program your habit. The food industry has a vested interest in you continuing to eat just as you always have. The food industry makes a *lot* of money by selling you cheap, unhealthy products, so they're going to do everything they can to get you to buy their stuff. They will launch marketing campaigns that are specially designed to please your senses so you'll want to buy what they're selling, and they'll concentrate flavors that get you hooked on their goods. They will lower prices by reducing quality, then reduce quality yet again in order to cut costs.

Now, instead of giving your money to the big food conglomerates, you're going to start buying your food from conscientious suppliers who bring you real, nutritious foods.

Remember what we said about energy balance in Chapter Three? Good nutrition will support the energy balance that optimizes your body composition. Your body composition is an important contributor to your health. If your energy balance favors energy conservation and weight gain, you will become less healthy. Obesity may follow, along with the many chronic diseases that accompany it. If you are having a problem with excessive body fat, then you have a problem with your energy balance. Remember that your energy balance and body fat regulation is hormonally regulated. We want to approach eating in a manner that supports normal hormonal function. Restoring hormonal balance is necessary for long term weight control.

Energy balance has many influencers, but your nutrition is a major one. Although we emphasize the importance of food sourcing, eating too frequently and overeating are still the predominant sources of excessive body fat. As explained in Chapter three, eating frequently increases insulin, which increases obesity. Also, eating foods that trigger inflammation negatively impacts your energy balance. You must learn how to eat the portions of food consistent with your energy demands. Too much energy coming into your body will send a fat storing message. You must send your body the right messages. Food is information to your underlying physiology. Too much of it sends a message to your body that will likely result in a response you find undesirable.

However, remember that too little food over a sustained period will also not provide the results you are looking for. We do not want you to under-eat except when applying fasting protocols or using our 9-week weight loss program. In those cases, it is not truly undereating. Brief periods of lower food consumption will have a therapeutic benefit for you.

Your nutrition plan ultimately must be individualized. There is no "one best diet" for everyone. Your body has the ability to perform well in a variety of different nutritional conditions. Your body can convert any primary nutrient into energy. There are examples from around the globe of very healthy populations who eat all kinds of different diets. Some are primarily fat, others primarily carbohydrates. You can be healthy whether you eat mostly meats or mostly vegetables, mostly fats or mostly carbohydrates. In the end, you need the nutrition plan that supports your health, maintains your energy balance, and is sustainable for you. If it is not sustainable for you, then it is not a good plan for you. We do provide some guidance to get your body moving in the right direction, but for the rest of your life, you will determine the nutritional approach that works for you.

What are the common attributes of healthy nutrition?

- Healthy nutrition involves you caring about your food and eating.

- Healthy nutrition involves food quality and sourcing.

- Healthy nutrition is comprehensive, reducing nutritional deficiencies.

- Healthy nutrition helps control appetite and how much you eat.

- Healthy nutrition catalyzes physical activity.

- Healthy nutrition involves feeding and fasting

- Healthy nutrition involves proactive stewardship of the environment

OUR EATING HABITS CHANGED— AND OUR HEALTH DECLINED

The food industry has been shaping the eating habits and food policy in this country for a couple of generations. Our entire understanding of food and nutrition has been influenced by an industry that is primarily focused on making money rather than providing healthful nutrients to the population. That industry is also intimately involved in designing and running the studies that are used to shape nutritional guidelines and health objectives. In other words, these companies have succeeded at influencing practically every aspect of how we buy and eat food.

Meanwhile, for the first time in a century, life expectancy in this country has begun to *decrease* thanks to a bevy of diseases that are linked to obesity, including heart disease and diabetes.[2] Consider the astonishing fact that almost one in every five American children (17 percent) is obese, and nearly 6 percent of children are *extremely* obese.[3] Medical journals are now reporting that obesity among adolescents may be the greatest threat to our health as a nation. This is a profound and urgent problem. We are creating a disordered metabolism in our children. The longer they have a disordered metabolism, the harder it will be to correct in the future. We would not give our children cigarettes if they asked for them. Why are we giving them minimally nutritious and highly addictive substances to fuel their bodies? This does not make sense. It is okay to have dessert occasionally,

---

2   Ludwig, David, "Lifespan Weighed Down by Diet," JAMA, 315, no. 21 (2016): 2269-2270.

3   Ogden C.L. et al., "Trends in Obesity Prevalence Among Children and Adolescents in the United States, 1988-1994 Through 2013-2014," JAMA, 315, no. 21 (2016): 2292-2299.

but not for every meal.

In developing this nutrition program to help my patients reverse the awful trend toward obesity and regain their health, I rooted through all the medical literature I could get my hands on—and I spent a lot of time studying what actually worked, and what didn't, for my own patients. In all that research, I realized something very important: obesity was not the root problem.

The root problem, which underlies our obesity and all its related diseases, is a system of habits. These habits trigger hormonal responses that ultimately cause obesity. Over a few generations in this country, we've developed habits that are now literally killing us. When we consume certain foods in excess quantity or excess frequency as a regular habit—as so many of us do—we're poisoning ourselves.

The situation has gotten so bad that the pharmaceutical companies are now coming out with drugs to inhibit the euphoric feeling you get from eating the unhealthy foods that have been specifically engineered to give you that euphoric response. One particular drug, which costs about $200 a month, has been very effective in helping some people tackle the psychological challenge of giving up their favorite junk foods. I prescribe this medication to many of my patients as part of a comprehensive weight loss plan, and it often does help them. Recently, a bariatric specialist came to my area to speak about the power of this particular drug. Though I was unable to attend, someone from my office went. During the Q&A session, a nurse practitioner raised her hand and asked about how patients can transition off the drug once it has been effective for them. What was the speaker's response? That patients *don't* transition off the drug—that, in essence, they remain on a $200-per-month prescription for the rest of their lives. If I had been there, I would have liked to mention the overwhelming research that shows we absolutely *can* rewire our brains, and that we don't need prescription drugs for the rest of our lives in order to do it.

I hope it now makes sense to you why I've so heavily emphasized habit in this book, and why I'll continue to do so through each chapter. We *must* look closely at our habits and begin to ask ourselves: Do I enjoy these foods so much that it's worth being chronically ill? Am I going to continue taking all these medications to deal with the symptoms of diseases that are caused by the foods I'm putting in my body, or am I going to choose something different for myself? Why would I choose an approach to nutrition that is making me sick? Is the discomfort you experience from chronic diseases and poor health less than the discomfort of change? It should not be.

This chapter and this book, and the philosophy in which they're grounded, are about helping you to make new choices to change your habits—permanently.

THE SIMPLE WISDOM IN BECOMING AWARE OF WHAT AND HOW YOU'RE EATING

It wasn't very long ago that the act of eating took a lot more time and attention than it does today. Before processed foods were widely available, food had much more texture and fiber. It actually took time and effort to chew. If you were eating vegetables, grains, and meats that came right off a farm, you couldn't possibly eat a big meal in a couple minutes while also multitasking, because it would have been dangerous. You'd risk choking to death. So mealtime was something of a ritual. It was a time to appreciate the sustenance you were putting into your body. It was often a time to gather as a community.

In recent times, though, we've become accustomed to wolfing down a twelve-inch sub sandwich, a bag of chips, and a soda in a matter of minutes while looking at our phones at the same time—and then we immediately return to whatever we were doing before the meal. It's possible to do that now because our food doesn't have the kind of texture it used to have. We can eat quickly, and we can do so while barely noticing what it is we're eating. We live in a time in which the cost of food, the availability of food, the textures of foods, and the demands of our busy lives are such that we don't take time to pause and eat. We don't stop to enjoy the flavors and textures of what we're consuming.

Then there is snacking. We do not need to snack. There is emerging evidence that the major contributor to our obesity epidemic is our increased frequency of food intake. We described this in detail in Chapter Three. Continual eating triggers continual insulin, which triggers continual fat storage. The only beneficiaries of our snacking habit are the corporations of the food industry, which sell us the food, and the pharmaceutical companies that sell us the drugs to treat the diseases caused by our dysfunctional eating. We have to learn how to lengthen the intervals between our meals and to tolerate occasional periods of fasting.

When food is abundant, as it is in our time, we should not be arranging our days around food. Our day should be spent making progress towards our goals. We should be thinking about what we can accomplish with the time we have. That could include rest as well as activity, but we should be thinking about our purpose, not food. Food is supposed to support our efforts at living purposeful lives. We should not be worried about what we are going to eat. There is no risk that you will not be able to find food. In times of food scarcity, we would naturally think a lot about food, because food is necessary for life. We would eat whenever we had the opportunity. We do not live in a time of food scarcity. The food manufacturers are competing with one another to see who can sell you the most food.

There are medical consequences associated with the way we eat. Your body sends certain signals to your brain that tell you to stop eating when you've consumed enough food—but those signals get scrambled as a result of our modern habits. The first signal comes simply from chewing and swallowing; that tells your brain that you're taking in nutrition. But chewing and swallowing quickly, instead of slowly and deliberately, alters that signal. Just chewing and swallowing will initiate hormonal responses in your body.

Then there's the way your midsection swells when you eat. As your stomach distends, your body sends another signal to your brain, this time telling you that you're full. That's supposed to keep you from overeating. And yet another signal comes as a result of your body actually detecting and absorbing nutrients. That sends a hormonal response that again tells your brain that you've eaten enough.

But eating quickly affects these signals, too. Your brain likely won't get the message until long after you've consumed your twelve-inch sandwich, chips, and soda—even if your body had enough when you were only halfway through.

Also, processed foods have poor nutrient density. We end up eating a large portion of food containing excessive calories but actually get very little nutrition from these foods. Consumption of nutrient-dense whole foods from natural sources actually causes greater satiety and reduces overeating. Eating nutritious foods is a natural appetite suppressant.

Consider this very different approach. Imagine eating unprocessed foods that have more texture and fiber than what you can get at a fast-food restaurant. And imagine taking the time to chew them and swallow deliberately. In between bites, perhaps you also take sips of water. The chewing and the swallowing, the gradual filling up of your stomach, the hydration, and the nutrients reaching your system all give your brain the opportunity to correctly process the signals that your body is sending it. Then your brain responds when you've eaten the appropriate amount by turning off your hunger. As a result, you actually *want* to stop eating.

Before we get into which foods to eat and which to avoid, there's a very important lesson in all this. The first step of this nutrition program is to give yourself more time for your meals. When it's time to eat, stop whatever you're doing and focus on eating. If possible, sit down with your family. Take smaller bites and chew slowly. Notice and appreciate the different flavors and textures in your food. If possible, try to chew each bite twenty-five times. Just experiment with chewing more and experiencing your food more. This improves satiety and also reduces gastroesophageal reflux and other digestive issues.

You'll probably find that you enjoy your food much more, and you'll give your brain the time it needs to recognize when you've taken in the necessary nutrients. Your brain will signal that you should stop eating when you've had enough.

Also, when you do not have the time to eat properly, you will learn how to just not eat. Your body will be fine. Once hunger no longer frightens you, you will have the power to choose skipping a meal until you have the time to eat what is actually good for you.

The notion that you should never miss a meal is completely false. We have to correct our thinking about this. You are better off not eating than actually eating much of what we call food these days. You will actually have less energy by eating an unhealthy meal. You will direct blood flow to your gut and away from your brain. You will spike your insulin. You may trigger inflammation. If you skip the meal, you will feel briefly hungry, but this will pass. You will retain your energy and avoid the negative consequences of consuming unhealthy foods.

Of course, if we ever actually enter into a period of famine in which food is unavailable to you for an extended period of time, I will modify this advice. I doubt that will happen in the near future. For now, learn how to manage your hunger. We will talk more about this below.

BUILDING NEW HABITS, ONE FOOD AT A TIME

Your current habits and eating patterns might favor certain flavors over others. Most likely, you're currently oriented toward foods that taste sweet and rich. But it's actually quite possible to begin to enjoy different flavors and textures, and eventually to shift your preferences in a different direction.

Right now, you might have an aversion to foods that have a trace of bitterness to them, such as leafy greens. If you were reared on foods that are very sweet and/or heavily fattened, your taste buds might find such bitterness unpleasant. But by incorporating the wisdom of the last section—the notion of slowing down your meals and chewing and swallowing more deliberately—you might be surprised at what you discover. You might find that you really like foods that you always thought you didn't.

As you begin to eat unprocessed, textured foods, start to build a positive habit by giving yourself specific reminders as you do so. Remind yourself that you're eating what's good for you—that you're eating what your body *wants*. Remind yourself that the flavors and textures you taste are delivering important nutrients, vitamins, and minerals that will give you energy, and that these are things you've been missing. Remind yourself that those nutrients will give you the energy you need and that they'll reduce pain and inflammation.

Then call to mind an image of the healthy version of yourself that you're striving for. Begin to develop an association between those healthy foods and that positive, healthy self. The more you can create a positive emotion around healthy foods, the more your body will crave them, because that positive emotion will function as a kind of reward. Make sure that you're not thinking to yourself as you eat nutritious foods that you *have* to eat them because your doctor said so. That negative association will undermine your progress.

This process of thinking positively about healthy foods is very important for achieving your goals—because a lot of what sits on grocery store shelves is *not* healthy, and reaching the good health you desire for yourself is going to take a lot of commitment. It will require effort in the form of retraining your brain. But if you keep at it, eventually you won't be tempted by the unhealthy foods that might have been your staples.

You're also going to help keep yourself from being tempted by intentionally developing some negative associations around the foods that are practically poisonous to you. Fast foods, processed foods, sugar-filled "nutrition" bars that claim to be healthy—you have to begin to see all of these things for what they are: toxic to your health.

These foods are actually nutritional stressors. This means they actually create stress for your body rather than providing healthy nutrients. Think about how exposing yourself multiple times a day to these foods is making you sick and tired. It may be happening slowly because our bodies are amazingly resilient. But eventually, your body's defenses and detoxification systems are overwhelmed by the daily exposure to these nutritional stressors. Eventually, these foods will cause diseases.

I want to emphasize for a moment that our bodies are well designed. They are designed to be very healthy. We are designed to live long and healthy lifespans. It is not normal to have diseases. Diseases only develop when the body is exposed to disease causing agents over a sustained period of time. These agents include environmental toxins, polluted water and air, drugs and alcohol, parasites, chronic unmitigated stress, nutritional deficiencies, and repeated exposure to nutritional stressors. It is *not* normal for us to be sick. We are designed for good health. It is especially abnormal for our children to be chronically sick.

Imagine for a moment that you're feeling very hungry. Let's say you're driving around in your car. You have a lot of appointments and you're very busy. But since you're hungry, you pull into a convenience store to grab a snack. Now let's say that the only things on the shelves of this convenience store are some household products: jugs of bleach, bottles of Windex, and pesticides for your lawn. No matter how hungry you get, you'd never select a bottle of pesticide and guzzle it.

That's how you've got to begin to see those processed foods. When you eat manufactured foods that are full of artificial fats and refined sugars, you are potentially harming your body. You don't vomit the way you would if you tried to drink pesticides or bleach—but your body does respond over time. You gain weight. You have no energy. You feel heavy and slow. Inflammation increases. All of these are potential effects of regularly ingesting unhealthy processed foods.

Remember this when you find yourself craving an unhealthy snack. Stop and tell yourself that it could be making you sick. You've got to use your higher-level thinking to remind yourself of the good health you truly desire and then steer away from the unhealthy mass-produced products masquerading as food.

I know that I'm using very strong language here. I'm not suggesting that there's an evil scheme in which the food companies are trying to poison you. But I am suggesting that this is business as usual in our country. These companies have found that we enjoy artificially sweet and rich foods, so they supply them to us. But the truth is that those foods are unhealthy. We've got to stop asking for them, by refusing to spend our dollars on processed foods that undermine health.

In fact, we never should have craved those foods in the first place. We never should have craved heavily sweetened and fattened foods with dyes and preservatives. But scientists in the food industry discovered that when we ate those things, they triggered an incredibly powerful reward response in our brains. This has a lot to do with the way we are wired. For most of human history, finding food was an energy intensive process. Our brains are wired to seek out sugary and fatty foods. Specifically, our brains will crave and overeat foods with salt, sugar, fat, and glutamate (meaty flavors). Also, we are designed to binge eat when we can. This design works fine when food is fibrous and nutrient dense.

But in our time, we've become habituated to eating food that cannot possibly benefit our bodies. Each time you find yourself reaching for something processed and unhealthy, remind yourself that it's poison, and turn away.

WHEN BEING BUSY MAKES IT HARD TO EAT WELL

I've had plenty of patients see great results from following the nutrition plan in this chapter, only to get derailed when life gets busy. Between work and family, they have so much going on that they just can't stop and take the time to purchase and prepare healthy foods. One day they find themselves so hungry that they end up just grabbing a sugary energy bar, even though they know it's unhealthy. They bite into it, and it tastes so darn good, and it was so easy. Soon they're giving in now and then, more and more frequently choosing those unhealthy foods just the way they used to, and very quickly, they're back where they started.

That's why *preparedness* is a crucial part of this program. Preparedness means taking a little time each week—maybe on Sunday, or whenever you can spare an hour or two—and going to the local grocery stores, or the local co-op, or the farmers' market. Think in advance about what food you're going to need for the entire week. Break it down into days. What will you eat each day? Then buy all of that food in advance and have it ready for each day, so that the busyness of life doesn't derail you from your goals.

That includes being prepared for the worst. When you have no time at all and you find yourself really hungry, what can you snack on that's consistent with your health goals? The tables at the end of this chapter will explain that. There are certain nuts and other foods that will become your go-to nutrition sources when you're in a bind. And then you have to make sure that you have them available, well ahead of the time when you'll need them. When you become truly hungry, a nutritious snack will satisfy you until you have time to find a healthy meal. Learning to fast will also help.

Imagine standing in that convenience store where the only things on the shelves are household chemicals. Instead of getting a snack, you just drink some water. Then you walk out the door and go on your way. You would rather be a little hungry than sick.

THE ONLY FOOD GROUP YOU HAVE TO ELIMINATE ISN'T A FOOD GROUP AT ALL

In the tables at the end of this chapter, you'll find a list of foods and a sample nutrition plan. It doesn't involve you cutting out any single food group, like carbs or natural sugars. But you *will* have to give up the foods that are toxic to your body. For the rest of your life, as much as possible, you've got to stop consuming poor-quality industrialized foods: processed grains, refined sugars, genetically modified produce, hydrogenated oils, industrialized vegetable oils, the dairy products full of additives (dairy can be good for you from the right sources), products that are full of preservatives, and artificial sweeteners. All of it needs to go. These foods are not going to give you health. They take it from you. It may take time to make this happen, but it does have to happen.

If you're unwilling to do this, then our approach may not work for you, and unfortunately, you're going to continue to struggle with the same health issues that brought you to this book in the first place. Whether it's your fatigue, your obesity, your diabetes, your chronic inflammatory diseases, your IBS, or your chronic indigestion, stop for a moment and think: are your favorite foods worth it?

I do understand that this approach might sound extreme. And in a sense, it *is* extreme. Compared to the way our country eats today, the nutrition plan in this chapter represents a sharp change of direction. Look at it another way, though, and it's what your great-grandparents would consider common sense. You're going to limit your diet to the way we ate a couple of generations ago, before the explosion in health problems that we're experiencing today.

It is okay to take your time while making these changes. There are many influencers of how you approach nutrition. The cost of food, availability of healthy foods, convenience, time, and many other variables have an impact on how we choose our foods. We want you to have long term success. It is okay if the process of changing your food sources takes a bit of time. It is okay if you cannot change everything. Any positive changes you can make will improve your health. The more of this you can do, the more you can improve your health and well-being.

To help you make this leap to a different way of eating—and to a different way of thinking about the food that nourishes you—you'll also find a list of extra resources at the end of this chapter. These are resources that explain how industrialized foods are processed and the history of the industry. Having that information will help you understand why your diet is making you sick; that, in turn, will help you to take better care of yourself. It's beyond the scope of this book to give a complete overview of that information, but I'm going to offer just a bit of background here.

Picture a big, shiny apple sitting in a display at the grocery store. When you think of an apple, you probably think *healthy*. You might even picture the orchard in which the apple grew, and imagine it ripening in the sunshine.

But in our modern era, most apples at the grocery store are the product of industrialized processes. In order to increase the crop yield—and to reduce damage from pests, cut down the time it takes to get the product to the consumer, and limit the amount that spoils along the way—the agricultural industry uses a ton of chemicals.

That apple gets picked before it's ripe. Later, the apple goes through a "gassing" process in which it's covered in still more chemicals, this time to activate the molecules in the fruit that turn it an appealing color and make it plump and appetizing. Then, in its final stage, it gets coated in wax to make it prettier and more appealing to the consumer eye.

When you select that apple from the display in the grocery store and take it home and bite into it, you'll find that it's extremely sweet—much sweeter than an apple grown in a local orchard without all those chemicals. It's also much larger, meaning that it contains two or even three times as many calories from sugar. An apple grown organically at a local orchard looks and tastes very different. It's not only smaller and less sugary, but it isn't so perfect or round. But it is truly nutritious for you.

Part of this chapter's nutrition guidelines include a list of the produce that you absolutely have to buy organically, as well as a list of those that you can get away with buying conventionally. The underlying message, though, is to begin to seek out and purchase foods grown through natural methods. That often will mean buying fruits and vegetables sourced from your own area, because the foods that come from far away have been sprayed with chemicals to prevent spoilage. What's more, the locally sourced foods have been allowed to ripen on the vine or in the ground. When fruits and vegetables finish maturing in that way, they're more nutritious, because they've been allowed to absorb vitamins and minerals from the ground during their final ripening.

All of that had to do with just your fruits and veggies. Let's take a second to consider the more heavily processed foods, which typically contain artificial fats. You've probably heard the term "partially hydrogenated vegetable oil." Hydrogenated oils, which were originally intended to improve our heart health by reducing consumption of saturated fats, represent one of the worst experiments in the history of the food industry. Hydrogenated oils are toxic. We should never eat them.

As these oils are produced, they're held in big storage tanks, then transported across large distances. When we eat them, we're actually consuming heavily contaminated oils that have unnatural ratios of omega fatty acids. Eating them contributes to obesity and painful inflammation, and we *don't* get the healthy fats that our bodies actually need and want.

Foods are now required to carry labels about whether or not they contain trans-fats, which are in hydrogenated oils. But the food companies are very savvy about using these fats in small enough quantities, and manipulating the serving sizes, so that they come in just under the FDA threshold for the required label. You need to start reading the ingredients on the foods you buy in order to check for hydrogenated oils—and then avoid them like the plague.

Consider this fact about the nature of the fats found in our modern western diet. Omega-3 fatty acids are known to be anti-inflammatory and anti-thrombotic. This means they have the potential to reduce the inflammatory and blood clotting processes in your body. Omega-6 fatty acids, on the other hand, have the potential to increase the inflammatory and blood clotting processes in your body. Our historic diet results in the consumption of a ratio of Omega-3s to Omega-6s in a range of about 1:1 to 4:1; in other words, the person who follows our diet is unlikely to consume more than four times as much Omega-6 fatty acid than Omega-3. By contrast, the modern western diet, with its synthetic and industrialized fats and low-quality animal products, results in consumption of about a 16:1 ratio of Omega-6s to Omega-3s. Think about what that does to your health. The *British Medical Journal* recently published an editorial citing this fact as an issue of global economic justice, given that people who live in poverty have access only to these unhealthy, poor-quality foods.

Instead of processed fats, you're going to start eating natural, healthy fats such as organic olive oil and coconut oil, and nuts and avocados. You'll find specific guidance on which foods are healthy, and which aren't, at the end of this chapter.

Unfortunately, you can't trust *any* of the labels on the front of packaged foods; you *have* to turn them over and look at the ingredients. Consider this perverse example of how our country's food labeling system distorts the concept of "healthy." A product called Kind Bar is made from completely natural ingredients: nuts, berries, some natural dark chocolate, and some cinnamon. It has no refined sugars, hydrogenated oils, or anything processed at all. But because these Kind Bars contain nuts, which are high in saturated fat, the FDA forbids the manufacturer from printing the word "healthy" on the front label.

Meanwhile, right beside the Kind Bars in the grocery store aisle, you'll find a popular high-protein snack bar from a major food company that *is* allowed to carry the label "healthy." But what are the ingredients in that one? You guessed it: artificial sweeteners, artificial flavors, protein added in the form of a powder, hydrogenated oils, and preservatives and other chemicals. The fact that this processed snack bar is certified as healthy and the natural product is not shows the perversity of our system. You will have to educate yourself and then follow your own guidelines rather than relying on any of the labeling at the store. Our website has a short video explaining how to read and understand food labels.

I know that all of this may at first seem intimidating. You might feel afraid that you're going to make mistakes and eat the wrong things and thereby compromise your health. Don't worry, and please don't feel afraid. If some of these types of foods accidentally leak into your diet as you get the hang of this new nutrition plan, that's okay. You just don't want to contaminate yourself with these foods on a regular basis.

I'm also not suggesting that you should never eat at restaurants. You can eat out. Your just have to be mindful about the foods you order and what restaurants you visit. Our web hub has some guidance about how to eat healthy when eating out.

You might be wondering about the cost of all this. Are natural foods going to cost you more money than the regular stuff? Yes, they are. Organic produce costs more because it's more expensive to produce. You're also going to have to eat it more quickly once you've purchased it; it can't sit in the refrigerator for a week without shriveling, because it's not covered in stabilizing chemicals. But if you find yourself worrying about the cost or the inconvenience of more natural foods, remind yourself of the cost and discomfort of remaining sick. By comparison, natural foods are *much* less expensive. And as you grow healthier, you're going to spend a lot less money on medications and other healthcare expenses. That's money you can put toward your food budget.

CHOOSE NATURAL MEATS AND FISH

Our modern food system has developed industrialized processes for getting meats and fish to you as quickly and cheaply as possible—and the upshot is that we're consuming unhealthy animal products.

Consider the process by which livestock are raised and harvested. Animals are separated from their mother shortly after birth, placed in a crowded, unnatural environment with little or no exposure to the outdoors, fed unnatural foods, and injected with anything that will help them grow faster. They live their short, miserable lives in an environment that's unhealthy from a mental and physical standpoint. Remember that these are sentient animals; they can feel fear and dread. They know something's off. Then they're quickly turned into the plastic-wrapped product at your grocery store in order to turn a profit.

The result is meat that's pretty close to fake food. It bears little resemblance to meat from animals raised with natural methods. When animals grow naturally in their own environment, with their kin and on their own timeline, their meat becomes a healthy source of protein for you, with the right ratios of essential fatty acids.

The same thing goes for pigs and other types of livestock, as well as fish. Farm-raised fish eat food that isn't really fish food, so that they'll fatten up quickly. That's why they look different from wild-caught fish. Wild-caught salmon is a deep red, while its farm-raised counterpart is a weak pink.

So as you move into the nutrition program of this chapter, you've got to begin to shift your purchasing habits. If you're going to eat animal protein, then you need to choose products from animals that developed naturally. This new kind of meat will taste a bit different. It will be a little leaner, a little gamier, a little less fatty. It will be more expensive. You may end up needing to eat meat less frequently in order to afford the natural variety when you do buy it. That's not a bad thing; it's a sign that you're consciously shifting your food budget toward producers who care about the animals and about the quality of the product they're selling you. Make sure your seafood is "wild-caught". Make sure your beef and dairy are from "grass-fed" pasture raised cows. Make sure your chicken and eggs are from "pasture-raised" chickens. It is very important to pay attention to these details.

BETTER THAN THE "LOW-CARB" CRAZE: NATURAL STARCHES AND GRAINS

Your body can exist without starches. They are not an essential nutrient. Your body can make its own sugar from amino acids and fats. Proteins and fats are essential nutrients, while carbohydrates are not. However, just about every human civilization throughout history, with the exception of nomads, has had some form of starch or grain as its staple food. Although many of our popular diets would have you completely eliminate all starches from your diet, you do not have to. Also, there are some individuals whose genetics favor a higher carbohydrate diet. It is important to understand how to approach carbohydrates in your individualized eating plan.

Decades ago, before we became obese, people were eating breads, pasta, rice, and potatoes. They just were not eating them as frequently or in such large portions. If your sustainable eating plan includes carbohydrates, that's okay. You just have to understand the differences between processed starches and healthy starches.

From Chapter Three, you know that ketogenic diets are a great way of initiating weight loss, but also that in the long term, some individuals perform better with access to some carbohydrates as fuel. In that chapter, I described the way a diet that eliminates all carbohydrates and sugars and is low in calories might lead to rapid weight loss but might also result in people having very little energy and constantly battling hunger—and if those people go back to normal eating for a moment, they often gain back the weight they've lost. We also described how that is not due to ketogenic diet itself, but rather from undereating or other hormonal changes in the body.

It's also true that people experience weight loss plateaus when changing their diets. People who needed to lose forty-five pounds would lose thirty, and then no more. People who needed to lose eighty pounds would lose perhaps forty. We now understand what was happening. Their bodyweight and body fat percentage were being managed by neuro-hormonal signals. The use of long term low calorie diets was triggering a hormonal response that favored regaining the weight that was lost.. It was not the presence or absence of carbohydrates that was causing the issue, it was the ineffective approach to losing weight. Lowering carbs can help with weight loss. However, it is the overconsumption of calorie-rich and minimally nutritious foods that is preventing weight loss, not the carbohydrates.

You don't have to stop consuming starches and grains. That's not what's making you sick—not exactly, anyway. The problem is in the way those and other foods have fundamentally changed over time.

Consider that the wheat we eat today has been crossbred over and over and is harvested in a process that's very different from how our ancestors harvested. When you eat modern wheat products, you end up consuming a higher concentration of gluten than you would have before. That has led to some digestive issues that have made the term "gluten intolerance" a widely known concept.

But at the root of those digestive issues is not the gluten itself, but the fact that we're consuming foods that are from fundamentally altered sources. Our ancestors would reject what we now call wheat. At the end of this chapter, you'll have a list to help you choose the right starches and grains derived from healthy seeds. There is also a list of starchy tubers that are a healthy source of carbs.

Our processed grains have had most of the protein, fiber, fat, and nutrients pulverized out of them. What is left is a chain of simple sugars that quickly digests and quickly enters your bloodstream. This leads to a prompt insulin response. Our refined flours and processed grains are minimally nutritious for us and are significant contributors to insulin resistance and diabetes. You will need to consume starches that retain the fiber and other nutrients that Mother Nature put into them. Humans keep thinking we can engineer food better than Mother Nature. It is not true. We keep proving that our trying to outsmart Mother Nature almost always fails when it comes to food.

Also, improperly prepared grains and legumes are not fit for our digestive systems. In order to be able to digest these foods, they need to have been soaked, fermented, or sprouted. Non-GMO, non-processed, and properly prepared grains and legumes can be very good for us. Some individuals do not tolerate them well. But if you do, they can be a great source of energy and nutrients.

DIETARY SUPPLEMENTS—YEA OR NAY?

Many of my patients ask whether supplements will help them on their quest to be healthier. In particular, they tend to ask questions about supplements that are supposed to speed up your metabolism. Studies have shown that most of these don't really work—so be careful how you spend your money.

Certain supplements can be helpful if you have a vitamin deficiency or a disease, or if you take a medicine that affects your absorption of vitamins and minerals. In any of these cases, though, you should be in communication with your medical provider about which supplements are necessary and appropriate for you.

If you don't have a particular health problem that requires special vitamins, then you likely don't need any supplements at all. Instead, if you source your food well and eat a variety of healthy produce, you'll get all the vitamins and minerals your body needs. Then you can take all the money you saved by not buying those expensive supplements and put it toward your food budget.

However, there are some supplements that may help you. Those containing trace minerals, omega-3 fatty acids, phytonutrients and micronutrients, and others.

If you plan to follow a true ketogenic diet and actually maintain yourself in a continual state of nutritional ketosis (more information about nutritional ketosis is available at www.healthshepherds.com), then I do recommend certain supplements. It is beyond the scope of this book to teach people how to maintain a state of nutritional ketosis.

Our Health Shepherds web site has more information about supplements. I personally use a variety of food-based nutrient containing supplements on my fasting days. I provide a list of what I take on the web hub.

THE OMNIVORE'S FORMULA:
MORE PLANTS, FEWER ANIMAL PRODUCTS

It's important to strike the right balance in your diet between plant- and animal-based products. The American diet typically contains more animal products than are necessary or healthy.

There are a lot of misconceptions about how much meat is healthy to consume, and many people incorrectly believe that vegetarians don't get enough protein. In fact, you can become a vegetarian and get all of the proteins and vitamins and many of the minerals you need. If you've considered becoming a vegetarian, I would highly recommend it as a pathway toward regaining your health. A plant-based diet that is not high in sugar or processed grains is a very healthy option.

Another option is to take intermittent fasts from animal products. In other words, you can occasionally cut meat and/or other animal products from your diet for a set period of time. A nutrition professor has developed a two-week introductory program to help people explore a plant-based diet; you can find the curriculum at www.14dayhealthchallenge.com.

APPETITE CONTROL AND THE SKINNY ON FASTING

There are many experts who criticize our modern-day diet for the fact that we consume too much food too frequently. Their criticism is warranted. As you learned in Chapter Three, our tendency to snack continuously between meals makes it more difficult for us to use our stored fatty acids as fuel which contributes to weight gain and obesity. This makes it much more difficult when people do attempt to lose weight.

Periodic fasting—that is, going for a set number of hours without food—can be healthy for most individuals. Our bodies are designed to tolerate fasting and perhaps even thrive during fasting conditions. Fasting is a learned skill, especially given how often we have been told to eat. There are some who should not fast. Children and pregnant woman should not fast. Those with hypoglycemia should not fast. Individuals on multiple medications or insulin can fast, but they should be closely supervised by a physician. However, the vast majority of us can fast and *should* fast.

I want to make sure you understand that I am referring to any interval of time when you are not eating as fasting. Fasting can involve longer periods of time without food or just a few hours. If the word "fasting" sets off alarm bells in your mind, it should not. Fasting is just spacing your meals out. It is not hard. Eating a reduced calorie diet every day is hard, but fasting is not.

I emphasize fasting so much because we have become unbalanced in our approach to eating. Often when I suggest fasting to a patient, they will stare at me in disbelief. They immediately think I have suggested something unsafe and extreme. I then have to spend significant time explaining how their body works. Once I do, they always end up saying "that makes sense". Of course it does. Your body is well designed to provide you energy when you are not eating. It has ample fuel available, even for extended periods of time. Your body likes to fast. It is your mind that resists fasting. I hope to help you change your mind so you can begin to experience the benefits of allowing your body periods of fasting.

I am going to provide some basic information about fasting in this chapter. It is enough information for you to begin to incorporate fasting into your own dietary routine. However, for those of you who want to know more about fasting, we will list resources on our web hub that can expand your understanding of fasting.

I am trying to keep the information in this book as straightforward and action-oriented as possible. In my experience as a physician, I have found that most of my patients just want me to do the research for them and provide them with an understandable action plan. Most of my patients do not want to read lengthy books on nutrition, metabolism, obesity theory, exercise science, and other medical topics. They have their own interests, hobbies, professions, and areas of expertise to read about and research. They trust me and count on me to provide them with their individualized proactive health plan. The proof is in the pudding. If they feel good, and their health biometrics look good, then what we are doing together is working.

However, if you are one of those individuals who likes to read everything about whatever you are doing, then we will list plenty of resources for additional study on our web hub in each habit category. In my experience, too much information can prevent people from starting something helpful for them. Researching a nutrition plan can actually become a substitute for implementing a nutrition plan. We discussed this in our chapter on self-control. At some point, you have to start doing whatever needs to be done.

In many cases, it is not what you need to start doing, it is what you need to stop doing. In fact, behavioral research suggests that people are more likely to change when they are given a *pro*scription rather than a *pre*scription. Telling them not to sit on the couch and watch television is more likely to get them up and moving than telling them to get up and move.

That is what is great about fasting. We are not giving you something else to do, we are giving you something *not* to do: eat! Fasting does not cost money. Fasting does not involve food preparation, shopping, or food selection. Fasting allows you to use your own stored energy for fuel. Fasting takes your mind off of food so you can focus on productive activities. Fasting is perhaps the easiest habit to adopt if you are willing to give it a try. It is also one of the most effective ways to improve your health and weight.

As we discussed in Chapter Three, fasting leads to an increase in your metabolic rate, and it facilitates fat adaptation, the process of your body using fat for energy. Fasting does not cause muscle wasting; it protects against it. Fasting can be used for long-term weight loss without slowing your metabolism. It does not make you tired, achy, depressed, or trigger a state of brain fog the way long-term daily calorie restriction does. There are some short-term challenges when learning to fast, but they are short-term; they don't last long. Fasting enables you to discern true hunger from false hunger. Fasting gives you control of your hunger and allows you to align your eating behaviors with your actual metabolic needs. Fasting helps you to enjoy food rather than bingeing on it. Fasting helps restore a functional relationship to food. Fasting has been used for thousands of years for the purpose of improving health. Every major religion prescribes fasting as a method of deepening faith. I think you get the point, fasting is good for you and safe for you.

Fasting is safe for almost everyone. There is a lot of mythological thinking about fasting that is not based on any evidence. I will not go into the details in this chapter. However, if you have heard that fasting is extreme or unsafe, then that is incorrect. Most humans over all of human history have fasted. Over the past fifty years, food has been so over-marketed to us, and our public policy makers have been so influenced by food manufacturers, that it has been hard to learn the truth about fasting. Food manufacturers do not want you to learn fasting. They would like to continue to condition your eating behaviors towards eating a lot of the food they are selling. It is time for you to take back control of your nutrition and align your eating habits with your highest desires. Fasting will help you do that.

The discomfort you feel when you temporarily go without food is partly due to your body's inability to use your own stored fuel. Your hunger is not associated with your nutritional needs. It is a behavioral conditioning pattern. If you are overweight, obese, or diabetic, this should motivate you. Others that do not care for you, and who actually want your money, have purposely influenced your thinking to eat in a manner that keeps you overweight and sick.

Then others also seeking your money come to you and provide you with the solutions to the fact that you cannot lose weight and are unhealthy. They tell you to buy their program which will teach you how to eat less and move more. They will also sell you some supplements to help you reach your goals faster. If you do their program, it works. You lose weight and feel better. The supplements were probably a placebo, but perhaps the idea that the supplement helped you motivated you a bit. You feel better. Your friends and family tell you how great you look.

Then slowly, month by month, you find your way back to where you started, overweight and chronically sick. Perhaps you started overeating again and stopped exercising. Or perhaps you tried to maintain your healthy program but still regained the weight. Now everyone, including your doctor, suggests to you that you must be overeating and not exercising. They blame you for your obesity. You feel ashamed and guilty. Perhaps you give up. No one tells you that the program you bought was just a Band-Aid and the supplements were a placebo.

Meanwhile, your diabetes worsens and you are given a prescription for another medication. This medication will actually increase your insulin levels, causing you to gain even more weight. The cycle goes on and on. No one told you about the strong, accumulating evidence that low-fat, low-calorie diets slow your metabolism and ultimately fail to provide the long-term results you are hoping for. No one suggested you consider fasting or perhaps a ketogenic diet. That would be too extreme. However, it would probably work. If the current paradigm cannot produce the results you are seeking, it is time to look outside the paradigm.

The concept of intermittent fasting suggests that you can incorporate a particular rhythm into your weekly schedule. I recommend starting with just extending your overnight fast. Try to eliminate any evening snacking. After your dinner, try not to eat until your breakfast the next morning. Try to have at least a twelve hour interval every day where you are not eating. Then, once you are successful with that, start skipping breakfast. Yes, you heard me correctly: skip breakfast.

When we first wake up in the morning, we are in a natural fasting state. Your body's hormonal systems are actually providing you with the energy you need to get your day started. Your body has already provided for you what breakfast is supposed to provide. You are using your glycogen or stored fat for fuel. When you start your day by eating, you increase your insulin and turn off any potential fat adaptation that may be taking place.

Most people are not naturally hungry in the morning. The breakfast food industry has trained us to think we need food right away every morning. Not only that, most breakfast foods are full of processed carbohydrates and sugar; therefore, they increase insulin. I just checked the label on a box of cereal marketed as a breakfast food for kids. The primary ingredients were rice, sugar, hydrogenated vegetable oil and artificial dyes. There is no universe that exists in which this is part of a healthy breakfast. Any breakfast that would have been healthy is made unhealthy by eating this as part of it. We have been told that eating these foods first thing in the morning actually improves our metabolism. There is no proof of that. If you understand the basic physiology lesson from Chapter Three, you can now see through all of the misinformation about nutrition we are being provided.

To learn how to fast, start by just extending your usual overnight fast. Try to go twelve hours without eating. Then try to go fourteen and then perhaps longer. You can base this off of any meal you would like. If you prefer to fast after a morning meal then that is fine. Most just find it easier to extend the overnight fast. One protocol suggests we eat only during an eight-hour window each day. Provided you eat adequate amounts of food and make healthy choices, this can work. It is important to vary your approach to fasting over time. The body seeks homeostasis and will metabolically adjust to any regular feeding schedule.

For more information about fasting and more protocols for fasting, visit our web hub at www.healthshepherds.com. For now, I would like you to consider adopting a simple fasting protocol. I would suggest you vary the time of your overnight fast and try to get it between 14 and 16 hours if you are able. I would suggest one 24-to-36-hour fast per week. I personally do this as part of my routine. . It is okay to take your time learning how to do this. You don't need to be in a rush.

It can take a little time to adjust to fasting. If it becomes too uncomfortable, you should just break your fast and eat. It may take a month to start to really adapt to fasting. Usually, after one month of consistent fasting, the process becomes much easier. It does not take long to really start to enjoy how good you feel when you are fasting. Eventually, you look forward to fasting the way you look forward to feasting. I know that sounds crazy, but it is true.

Here are the reasons you should try to do this. A 24-hour fast will cut anywhere from 1800 to 2500 calories out of your weekly intake *without* slowing your metabolism. Even if you eat a little more than usual on the day after your fast, you still will have reduced overall calorie consumption substantially. A pound of fat is 3500 calories. For each day you fast, you will lose about a half pound of fat without slowing your metabolism. Longer fasts, 48 hours, will allow you to lose more fat each week.

On your non-fasting days, you will not calorie restrict. In fact, it is very important that you do not calorie restrict. Sustained calorie restriction leads to a slower metabolism. Fasting does not slow your metabolism. I want you to fast, but then eat normally on the other days. We will talk extensively about what I consider eating normally in the remainder of this chapter.

Making sure you eat adequate amounts of food on non-fasting days can be more challenging than you would think. Over time, learning to fast will give you so much control of your appetite, you will be tempted to eat less all of the time. You will be less hungry. If you are trying to lose weight, you will find you are able to control your appetite. You may think eating less every day will facilitate faster weight loss. It will not. You must eat normal portions of healthy foods on your non- fasting days.

If you want to lose more weight faster, then simply add in more fasting days or longer fasts. It is reasonable to fast every other day for an extended period of time if you need to lose a lot of weight. You would fast for 24 hours then eat normally for 24 hours. You would repeat this for as long as you need to lose weight. However, I would recommend working with your physician and closely monitoring your biometrics if you are going to fast this often. You can also train yourself to fast for 48 hours once a week and then eat normally the other five days. There are many different fasting schedules that can be adopted. If you are going to fast frequently then please review our documents on fasting on our web hub so you are aware of the few potential complications. Shorter fasts do not have any complications as long as you stay hydrated.

On your fasting days you should drink plenty of water. It is fine to have coffee and tea. You should avoid all sugars and artificial sweeteners as they raise insulin. One of the reasons fasting works is it lowers your insulin levels and facilitates fat adaptation. Artificial sweeteners raise insulin and interfere with this process. That is why diet sodas are not a solution. They still trigger insulin and contribute to obesity and diabetes. You can take a high-quality multivitamin on your fasting days. You can also have a cup of bone broth to replace salts. Our web hub has a suggested recipe for making your own bone broth. You can choose to drink only water, and that is perfectly fine. Your body can tolerate 24-48 hour fasts with only water without any problems. If you like, you can put coconut oil, MCT oil, or organic cream in your coffee or tea. This does provide some fat calories, but it will interfere minimally with the results of your fast.

Fasting is easy, but it is also a complex topic. It's beyond the scope of this book to teach you everything about fasting. However, it isn't hard to get started. Here is a summary of how to initiate fasting as part of your nutritional routine.

1. Extend your evening fasts by skipping breakfast. You may start a fast after breakfast or lunch if that works better for you.

2. Eat only two or three meals daily with no snacks in between.

3. Try to incorporate a 24-to-36-hour fast each week.

4. Do not force fasting into your life when conditions do not favor fasting (vacations, weddings, birthdays, etc.).

5. Stay well hydrated while fasting.

6. Do not overeat when breaking your fast. Start with a small meal or perhaps just a snack such as a handful of nuts.

7. Expect to experience hunger and some physical and emotional discomfort when you start. You must be prepared for this and determined to work through it. After a month, fasting becomes much easier.

8. If you experience severe hunger, nausea, dizziness, severe weakness or other intense physical symptoms, then go ahead and eat. Do not try to fast through intense discomfort. Just try again once you have recovered.

9. On your non-fasting days, eat normally. Do not under-eat on your non-fasting days.

10. Vary your rhythm of fasting. Experiment with different lengths and frequencies of fasts.

11. Make fasting a lifelong habit of health.

Think about what hunger is for a moment. It is supposed to be an important message to our brains that we should start searching for food. That's our natural survival instinct. For most of human history, hunger was an indicator to obtain more food. At the same time, for most of human history, once your brain received that signal to search out food, it would take a while before you actually found it. And during those intervening hours (or days), we humans would have to deal with the sensation of hunger.

The reason that we're capable of dealing with that sensation has to do with the physiology of hunger. Your body tells your brain to feel hungry *before* you've actually depleted your stored nutrition. That way, you've still got extra energy saved up to serve as fuel while you find more food. The early stages of hunger are not supposed to make you panicky or depressed. This would be maladaptive. It would be hard to use your brain properly to find food if you were in a state of near panic because of your hunger. Historically, you needed your brain and body to work well when it was time to hunt and gather food. We would not have survived as a species if periods of fasting caused bodily weakness and brain fog.

The situation is different in our modern times. Whenever we have the thought that it'd be nice to have some food, we can just go grab it and eat it. Food is all around us, all the time. What's more, we're surrounded by foods that have been specifically engineered to be habit-forming—which means we crave certain foods whether we're hungry or not. We crave sugar. We crave that yummy fat. We crave salt.

We also eat for reasons that have little or nothing to do with hunger or cravings. Sometimes we eat to break up a mundane part of our day, or to reward ourselves for finishing a task. Sometimes we eat for the social engagement, when we meet with friends to eat and drink. In all of these situations, we're not using food as a source of nutrition, which is the right and healthy way to approach food. Instead, we're using food to fulfill some other need.

Part of your road to good health involves understanding your own hunger. You're going to need to get comfortable with it in a way that you likely aren't right now, because you can no longer let your hunger dominate you. You cannot let it drive you straight to the behavioral response of eating. You're going to have to deal with your hunger to achieve your long-term goals.

Recall what you read in the previous chapter about your awareness and thinking. Start to become aware of what's driving your hunger; try to notice if you're feeling the inclination to eat because of boredom, or because you want comfort, or because you're actually hungry.

And when you begin to feel hungry, try to sit and simply observe the feeling. How does the hunger manifest in your body? Is it emotional, is it physical, or is it both? What exactly makes it so uncomfortable? Sit there and simply feel that discomfort. Remind yourself that you're not starving. You actually have enough nutrition stored in your body to last you weeks or even months.

As you consider the discomfort of hunger, ask yourself: Is this feeling of hunger more troubling than the fact that my body won't use its stored fatty acids as fuel, and it's instead telling me to go eat more?

Remember the idea of neuroplasticity. You have the ability to change the habits that are currently programmed in your brain. Right now, your habit is to follow that hunger signal and eat a snack. Instead, try consciously telling yourself a different message: you're bothered by the fact that your body won't release its fatty acids, and you don't want to eat a snack right now because doing so is counter to your goals. You want to reach your goals more than you want to snack.

Then see if you can take it one step further. As you experience the sensation of hunger, and as you feel the discomfort associated with it, try a new way of thinking about that discomfort. Think of the discomfort as a sign that you're making progress toward your goals. If you never feel hungry, you're probably never going to become healthy and lose weight. So start to think of that physical discomfort as the evidence that you're going to be successful. You *are* going to reach your goals.

If the discomfort is really too much—or if you feel a gnawing pain or nausea—perhaps try eating something very small that does not have sugar and drinking a glass or two of water. Eating and drinking a little bit sends a signal to your body that something's coming into the system, which should reduce the severity of your symptoms. Having a serving of water, sparkling water, tea, or coffee is a great way to reduce hunger while fasting.

Then try to bring yourself back to this idea that the hunger is the feeling of your success. It's the feeling of your fat cells protesting that they have to give up the goods that have been hurting you so badly for so long. Really focus on interpreting that hunger signal as something positive; it's the feeling of achieving your goals. And because it's positive, tell yourself that you want to dwell in that hunger as long as you can. You actually *want* to feel that discomfort for a longer stretch of time—because the longer you feel it, the closer you are getting to your goals. It's the feeling of success.

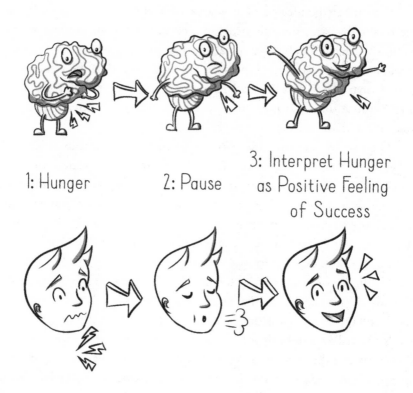

1: Hunger   2: Pause   3: Interpret Hunger
                                     as Positive Feeling
                                          of Success

I'm guessing that this approach to hunger will be entirely new to you. I've had patients who have gone to bariatric centers to lose weight and who have taken appetite suppressants and who have signed up for many different weight loss programs. In other words, they've tried just about every resource out there to help them lose weight—but no one has ever talked to them about controlling their appetites in the way that you just read.

I've had patients for whom this ends up being the most impactful part of the entire program. This idea of beginning to get comfortable with hunger, and then interpreting the discomfort as success, is a powerful strategy. It may be your key to changing your habits for the better—permanently.

You might also remember the concept of epigenetics from the previous chapter. You have the power to change your entire relationship to food, through strategies for the way that you think about both food and hunger, as we just discussed, all the way down to your genetic code. The type of foods you eat, and where they're sourced from, have a direct impact on your DNA.

The precise expression of your DNA involves a process called methylation, in which biochemical signals turn on or off the expression of certain genes. The foods you eat, and the specific vitamins and minerals that you consume—as well as any resulting inflammation in your body—all affect this process of methylation. If you eat a diet of healthy nutrients from natural sources, you'll reduce inflammation, improve the health of your DNA, and improve your metabolism.

Meanwhile, by consuming unhealthy foods and snacking a lot, you can shut down the portion of your DNA that boosts your metabolism. You are what you eat—and you also *eat* what you *are*. If you see yourself as vital and healthy, you'll end up eating foods that agree with that self-image. If you have a low self-esteem, you'll end up eating in a way that agrees with *that* image.

YOUR COMPREHENSIVE PROGRAM FOR GOOD NUTRITION

In the pages ahead, you'll find all the guidance you need for adopting eating habits that will be transformative for your health. This is a program of two or three meals a day with minimal snacking. You'll have to source your foods well and pay attention to how you put together your meals. You'll end up enjoying delicious food from natural sources.

You may lose a lot of weight initially. After that, your weight loss might be slow for a while; your body will give up some of its extra weight and then plateau, because it takes time for your brain to accept the new set point for your weight. But eventually, you're going to teach your brain that you have plenty of stored energy, and that your body is getting all the nutrients it needs. Eventually, your body will give up still more of that stored fat until at last you get back to your genetic baseline weight. Remember, for most of us, this genetic baseline will not likely provide six-pack abs. It will, however, provide you with good health and good energy.

It's also possible that you won't lose much weight, although if your body needs to, you probably will. If you don't lose weight but all of your biometric indicators improve—and if you feel good, and you feel re-energized, and your pain starts to go away—it may not matter that you didn't lose weight.

The important thing is that you have your energy and your health.

Of course, the proof is in the pudding. When you find that your food no longer makes you feel sick but rather gives you energy, and you find that your blood pressure and cholesterol and blood sugar and triglycerides have all improved, and you find that your body simply *feels* good, down to its muscles, bones, and joints, you'll know that you've finally found the health that was within you all along.

We use a variety of approaches to assist individuals with weight loss. There is no one best diet for everyone. I am going to outline several different approaches, and you should choose the one that is most likely to succeed for you. I have already discussed fasting as an approach to maintaining a healthy weight. I do recommend fasting for nearly everyone. For many people, that is all they need to do. Incorporate periods of fasting, and then source your foods well on non-fasting days and eliminate snacking. It can be that straightforward.

I also outline in this chapter an intermittent carbohydrate-restricted diet choosing from the foods we list. Many people find this approach very effective and sustainable. This allows for the so called "cheat days" which sometimes helps people psychologically when changing their eating habits. I do not like the concept of the "cheat day". I feel that phrase undermines the process and makes it seem like healthy eating is undesirable and something you are tempted to cheat on. However, if it helps you succeed in the long run, then use it.

I have also written a mini-book on how to adopt a truly ketogenic diet and maintain a state of nutritional ketosis. You can learn more about this on our website. There is much evidence to support nutritional ketosis as a method of reversing diseases and improving energy. I do not recommend going from a standard American diet straight to a ketogenic diet. It takes time to become fat adapted and then ketone adapted. It is much easier to train your body to become metabolically flexible in a gradual manner. For those who would like to experiment with becoming ketogenic, I recommend starting with a lower carb (100-150 grams daily) diet, and then once adapted to that, lower carbs further. These details are available on the web hub.

Nutritional ketosis is not starvation. The state of starvation is occurring when daily energy intake is insufficient to support daily energy needs. Starvation can occur while eating all carbs or all fats. Nutritional ketosis is simply switching to different sources of energy to support your cellular function. On ketogenic diets, you take in adequate calories, they just come from eating more fat and less carbohydrate. There is a lot of misinformation about ketosis on the internet. Many doctors do not understand the basic principles. Make sure to get your information from reliable sources. The books I list are evidence based resources.

We also have two versions of a low-carbohydrate, low-calorie eating plan that are accessible through our website. These are 9-week plans that initiate weight loss. The 9-week plans will not slow your metabolic rate provided you normalize your diet after the nine weeks.

Our programs are evidence-based medical bariatric nutrition plans. Our 9-week plans include a four-week detox phase, followed by five weeks of gradual broadening of food choices. These plans include weekly menus with all meals and snacks listed and specific portions of each food provided. If you choose to use one of our 9-week plans, you should know that the 800-calorie version is considered a very low-calorie diet and requires close medical supervision. The other involves a more moderate calorie reduction designed to induce fat adaptation. These plans are available as PDF downloads on the Health Shepherds website. The moderate plan is a 1,100-calorie-per-day low carbohydrate diet. This plan is safe for most individuals. However, if you have chronic medical conditions that are monitored by a physician, or if you take medications for medical conditions, I strongly recommend that you get permission from your treating physicians before following this plan.

More than likely, the plans outlined here will substantially reduce your intake of carbohydrates and sugars as compared to your usual diet. It will also be very important for you to maintain hydration while following our plans. If you take diuretic medications, diabetic medications, or use insulin, you will likely need your treating physician to make adjustments in the doses of these medications and monitor your blood work more closely while following these plans.

Typically, when we place patients on our 9-week program, we have them come to our facilities weekly for weigh-ins and blood pressure checks. We also ask about symptoms such as dizziness, nausea, change in bowel habits, fatigue, headaches, and any other changes in how they may be feeling. This gives us the opportunity to counsel them about strategies to increase the likelihood of success with the program and to minimize any unnecessary discomfort.

We've treated hundreds of patients with this program, and many of them have had great success. We've treated people with severe obesity and multiple chronic medical conditions. We've treated people with type 2 diabetes who completely reversed their condition as far as their blood tests are concerned.

The most significant issue that limits success is a lack of preparedness for what it will take to stick with the program. Sometimes, even when our patients really want to feel better, they are not quite ready to endure the discomfort that results from change. Our program is challenging; it's intended to be. This is not a short-term, quick weight-loss philosophy. Our program is designed to retrain your eating habits entirely. It's designed to improve your ability to tolerate hunger, resist cravings, and cultivate a genuine desire for authentic nutrition.

Ultimately, for many people, this is a form of detox from sugars and processed foods. It's worth noting that this program resembles the way we treat other types of addiction. Generally speaking, addiction treatment involves withdrawing the patient from the addictive substance and providing them with support and accountability. We sometimes use medications to help them tolerate the withdrawal process and to gain control over their addictive cravings. We then train them in a long-term methodology to avoid further addiction by understanding the cues and triggers that might lead to relapse.

Essentially, we're doing the same thing in this nutrition program. We withdraw our patients from sugars and excessive carbohydrates. We may use medications to help control their appetites during that time. We provide regular support and accountability. We then liberalize the nutrition plan while making sure the patient understands the potential cues and triggers that increase the risk of relapse into poor eating habits. Long term success requires a comprehensive approach, so if you choose to follow our nutrition plan, I strongly recommend working with a nutritionist, counselor, support group, medical office, or personal accountability partner to maximize your chances of success. The more support you have, the better your chance of success.

As you follow this program, you might start to notice how aggressively the food companies market their processed foods. You can't get away from it. You'll see it (and smell it) all over the place. You'll see how easy it is to overeat and to eat the wrong foods. You might feel like you're swimming against the tide to maintain your healthy habits.

If this happens, you'll need to remain positive about all this and re-member that you're doing what's right for your body, your mind, and your destiny. And as you do so, you'll become a positive influence for those around you who are trying to change their own habits.

The nine-week structured nutrition plans available on our website are quite Spartan. You'll probably feel that your choices are much more limited than those in your usual diet. Our goal is to gradually moderate the diet so that you have more choices, but to do so only after you have successfully induced weight loss and have begun to move closer to your goals. We'll gradually introduce fruits and other healthy sources of carbohydrates for those who feel they need these foods as part of their long-term diet.

Note that we will *never* suggest that you reintroduce processed carbohy-drates or refined sugars. Most individuals will ultimately allow these foods into their diet occasionally—but *only* occasionally. Sometimes, there will be celebrations, birthday parties, and holidays where you'll just eat what you want. These occasional indulgences eventually will be okay, as long as you adhere to a healthy nutrition plan most of the time. Indulgences should *not* be daily.

Once someone approaches personal weight loss goals, we start to indi-vidualize the program. Every person is different, and everyone will ultimately need his or her own nutrition program. Typically, we can gauge a person's best plan by monitoring the biometrics—weight and body composition—and how the person feels. Some individuals will do better by staying on a higher-fat, moderate-protein, lower-carbohydrate diet on a continual basis. Others will do better with a more balanced variety of foods.

The goal of the program is to give you the competency to determine the best nutrition plan for you. Provided you source your food well, you *will* be able to figure out what works for you. We'll provide some general guidance about how to structure your long-term plan, including lists of foods that you can eat liberally. (As an additional resource, consider pur-chasing *The Wild Diet* by Abel James. You can combine the comprehensive food-sourcing information in that book with the basic approach found in this chapter.)

We will list foods that should always be organically sourced and those that do not have to be. We will offer some suggestions for calculating the correct portions of different foods and for timing your meals. We hope to give you all the competencies you need to create your best long-term nutrition plan that supports your health and vitality; our ultimate goal is for you to be your own nutritionist.

You will discover what works for you by monitoring your weight, your energy, and your hunger. We want you to enjoy food and benefit from how it supports your health. We want you to eat freely and abundantly without having to constantly measure your portions. We want you never again to experience diseases or symptoms because of the food you eat.

Although we provide some structured guidelines, you are encouraged to make substitutions if necessary. You should not eat foods that are hard for you to tolerate or that cause inflammation or allergic reactions. You can substitute freely from the lists provided as long as you stay within the same categories; that is, substitute a fat for a fat, or a protein for a protein, etc. We will also encourage you to use spices to flavor your food, drink a lot of water, and perhaps use a high-quality fiber supplement (such as organically produced psyllium husk) to help with bowel regularity.

There will be many tips and tricks you can employ to help you succeed with this program. If you have a day where you slip up and revert back to your old eating habits, don't worry. Just start again. Try not to let those slip-ups escalate into poor eating habits for a full day or multiple days. Remember that once you enter ketosis, a meal of carbohydrates will break the cycle and you'll have to restart the process. Over time, you will become so aware of how poor-quality foods make you feel that you will have less and less desire to revert to old habits.

Just remember: don't give up because of one bad day. Keep trying. If you do, you will surely succeed

HOW TO USE THESE NUTRITIONAL GUIDELINES

- *Always* source your foods well. The guidelines below provide instructions for consuming only high-quality (and in many cases, organic) foods. This is essential.

- Use the food charts provided to design your meals by choosing one item from column A, as much as you want from column B, and one item from column C. Do this two to three times a day, and minimize snacking. Items in column B will promote satiety. To maintain adequate daily calorie intake, you may need to increase the portions of healthy fats from column C.

- You can substitute a smoothie for any meal; many people choose to have a smoothie in lieu of breakfast.

- If for some reason you must snack, then the best option is non-starchy vegetables and water, which will help fill you up without putting the wrong nutrition in your system. For other snack foods, choose from the list provided.

- Limit carbohydrate intake according to the instructions provided, and consume *only* the healthy carbohydrates that are listed below.

EATING PLANS

The following information is a summary of our principles for healthy eating. When combined with our movement plan, a regular meditation practice, and sufficient sleep, this nutritional approach will dramatically improve your metabolism, your energy, and your health.

Here's how it works. We provide you with a list of foods and instructions for how to combine them into two or three healthy meals each day. If you're trying to lose weight, we suggest that you minimize your consumption of carbohydrates. We're going to recommend that you follow an eating plan of limited carbohydrates for a certain number of days, then have one day where you can add back carbohydrates if you feel you need to. By reducing your carbohydrates and sugars, and replacing them with non-starchy vegetables and fats, your insulin levels will lower and fat adaptation will be facilitated. Also, by increasing your consumption of fiber, phytonutrients, and omega-3 fatty acids, you will lower inflammation, which will improve your metabolism.

Here is a suggested plan for turning on your body's fat-burning metabolism:

- low-carb for nine days, then consume carbohydrates on day ten; then,
- low-carb for six days, then consume carbohydrates on day seven; then,
- low-carb for five days, then consume carbohydrates on day six; then,
- find your own ratio of low-carb days to carbohydrate-loading

days. This ratio can be three to one, four to one, nine to one— in other words, any rhythm that works for you. If you find your weight loss is slowing, increase your number of low-carb days and be very particular about the carbohydrates you introduce on your carbohydrate days (whether it's a carbohydrate day or not, remember that you're avoiding *all* processed foods).

Once you transition to a long-term nutrition program, you may find that you can consume healthy carbohydrates daily. We recommend you choose from the list of healthy carbohydrates provided later in this chapter. You may also find that you need to continue a program of low carbohydrates and increase your consumption of healthy fats. I am a big advocate of diets that are low in carbohydrates, moderate in protein, and higher in healthy fats. Provided the food is from healthy sources, these types of eating plans can facilitate a healthy weight and control your appetite naturally. However, if you wish to consume more carbohydrates and fruits, choose from the healthy options we suggest.

I have personalized my own diet based on the results of my genetic testing, gut microbiome testing, and my biometric and nutritional blood results. I eat a higher fat, lower carbohydrate diet. My protein intake is moderate. Because of my genetics, I eat less saturated fat and more mono and polyunsaturated fats. I also fast a lot. Most days, I will not eat until late afternoon. This is not to lose weight. I just have more energy when I do not eat until later in the day. Eating redirects energy away from the brain and to the gut. I like to keep my energy directed outwards until later in the day when I can eat a lot of nutritious foods with my family. Once it is time to eat, I do eat. I do drink coffee and tea during the morning. Sometimes, I eat a handful of nuts if I feel I need to eat earlier in the day.

I find this rhythm works for me. I also try to cycle into a state of nutritional ketosis several times a year for about four to six weeks at a time. This is to promote metabolic flexibility and to provide my body with the long term health benefits of nutritional ketosis. I also have crazy good energy when I am in ketosis.

It is fine to use homemade smoothies or protein shakes if this helps you improve your approach to eating. This can increase your intake of healthy fruits and vegetables as well as protein by utilizing a high-quality protein powder. Smoothies are great as a meal replacement, and there are many ways that you can make them delicious and healthy.

Do *not* be fooled by mass-produced, pre-made meal-replacement systems. Most of the time, these will be made from poor-quality ingredients that are bad for you; most manufactured smoothie powders contain sugar, preservatives, and other unhealthy additives, and most protein powders do not contain the mix of amino acids your body needs. They may also contain too much soy, or they might be made from the milk of unhealthy cows.

I recommend you find a protein powder that has high-quality whey protein from grass-fed, pasture-raised cows. There are many healthy options for whey protein, so take some time to research the one you choose. You can find examples of these on our website in the nutritional resource section. If you cannot consume dairy, then choose a plant-based protein powder. Again, see our website for examples. Yes, this will be more expensive—and it's worth it.

For smoothies and all meals, we are trying to ensure that you have the right blend of high-quality protein, fat, and fiber, and a nourishing variety of key nutrients.

SAMPLE SMOOTHIE RECIPE

- 1 to 2 scoops of high-quality whey protein (or plant protein) powder. This should contain 15 to 25 grams of protein, fewer than 6 grams of carbohydrate, less than 2 grams of sugar, and ideally should contain some dietary fiber;
- 1 tablespoon of Chia or Flaxseed (grind the seeds) to add omega-3s;
- 1/3 cup or less of fruit: berries, cherries, pear, peach, melon, orange, apple, kiwi, banana:
- 4 to 8 ounces of your choice of liquid: water, unsweetened plain almond milk, unsweetened plain coconut milk, canned full-fat coconut milk, herbal tea, whole fat yogurt, or kefir;
- extras: avocado, coconut flakes, melted coconut oil, MCT powder or oil, 1 to 2 raw pasture-raised eggs, 1 ounce of nuts or 1 tablespoon of a nut or seed butter, 1 tablespoon flaxseed oil, spices, cocoa

powder, or stevia for sweetening.

- Enjoy your smoothie as a replacement for any of your three meals.

FOOD TABLES

◆ Instructions:

- Choose one food from the first column in a portion that fits in the palm of your hand. It is important to moderate your protein. However, if controlling hunger is an issue for you, then more protein may promote satiety.

- Choose as much as you want from the second column. Try to eat as many different vegetables as you can. These vegetables provide you with the fiber and phytonutrients your body needs. they can be cooked or raw. We have a handout on our web hub that describes different ways to make eating vegetables more enjoyable.

- Use the foods in the third column to season or for cooking. (Some of the items in Column 3 are in the foods from Column 1, such as the fat that comes with animal protein.) Once your appetite is regulated properly, you can begin to increase your intake from column 3. These fats are good for you, especially the omega-3 fats. You will have to monitor how your body responds to consuming more fats. However, if you feel good and are losing weight, then you can consume more from column 3. Fats naturally improve satiety and reduce hunger. You may need to moderate your saturated fat depending on your health history. If so, eat more of the mono and polyunsaturated fats.

- Maximize your omega-3 fatty acid intake. The foods highest in omega-3s from the tables below are flaxseed oil, salmon, mackerel, herring, sardines, tuna, halibut, trout, walnuts, walnut oil, chia seeds, Brussels sprouts, kale, spinach, broccoli, and cauliflower.

- Fiber, Fiber, Fiber. Increase your daily fiber intake by eating plants, seeds, nuts, and other fiber rich foods. Fiber is your best ally for controlling hunger.

Column 1: Protein	Column 2: Vegetables	Column 3: Fats and oils
eggs-pasture raised	arugula	These can be used for cook-
turkey	organic lettuces (bibb,	ing with high heat
beef	romaine, leafy greens,	grass-fed butter
chicken	etc.)	beef tallow
pork	collard or mustard	avocado oil
bacon	greens	Ghee
ham	swiss chard	peanut oil
lamb	kale	Cocoa Butter
duck	cabbages	organic coconut oil
goose	radicchio	almond oil
buffalo	radishes	macadamia nut oil
bison	bok choy	unrefined palm oil
venison	jicama	
salmon	leeks	for dressings and low-heat
tuna	okra	cooking
trout	spinach	cold-pressed extra virgin
flounder	sprouts (especially	olive oil
herring	broccoli)	sesame oil
sardines	cauliflower	flax oil for salad dressings
cod	broccoli	walnut oil for salad dressings
halibut	celery	cod liver oil
shrimp	brussels sprouts	avocados
scallops	eggplant	nuts (organic, no pre-fla-
clams	onion	vored or pre-salted), 1 to 2
crabmeat	mushrooms	ounces per serving
mussels	scallions or green onions	almonds, brazil nuts, maca-
oysters	snow peas	damia nuts, pecans, pili nuts,
lobster	squash (yellow, acorn,	pistachios
beef jerky	butternut, spaghetti)	almond butter
dry-cured meats such as	zucchini	coconut
salami	cucumber	cream cheese
other game meats	carrots (no more than	fish oils
tofu/tempeh	two daily)	flax seeds
edamame	artichokes	chia seeds
cottage cheese	hearts of palm	sunflower seeds
	jalapeno or other spicy	whole fat dairy*
	peppers	whole fat Greek yogurt*
	bell peppers: red, yellow	unprocessed cheese*
	and green	
	spirulina	*limit portions to once daily
	asparagus	
	watercress	
	sea vegetables including	
	seaweed	

◆ Fruits
Apples, blueberries, blackberries, raspberries, cherries, grapes, grapefruit, kiwi, mango, nectarines, oranges, peaches, plums, pomegranates, lemons, limes, melons

◆ Spices
Basil, black pepper, cardamom, chives, cilantro, cinnamon, cloves, garlic, ginger, parsley, turmeric, Himalayan pink salt, sea salt, others

◆ Beverages
Water and sparkling water—add lemon, lime, or cucumber, also teas and coffee

◆ Sweeteners (try to limit)
Dark local honey, coconut sugar, stevia (but limit use), cherry concentrate, blueberry concentrate, pomegranate concentrate (all fruit concentrates should be unsweetened)

◆ Snacks
Choose 1/2 to 1 cup of the non-starchy vegetables from the list above
Combine with 1/2 cup of organic hummus or 1 tablespoon of organic nut butter

1/2 cup of full fat organic Greek yogurt or organic cottage cheese
Combine with 1-2 teaspoons of raw honey or a palmful of organic berries

Small palmful of raw organic nuts: almonds, pistachios, cashews, Brazil nuts, walnuts, or pecans

Palmful of high-quality beef jerky with a glass of water

Not actually a snack, but they reduce appetite: chia seeds, coffee, tea, water

There are many healthy snack options, and our listed resources can teach you more. Remember that we prefer you not to snack between meals if possible.

◆ Desserts (limit intake while trying to lose weight)
Seasonal fruits, preferably from local sources. Whipped cream made from organic cream.

◆ Nuts and cheeses
Dark chocolate, organic and at least 70 percent cacao. A small portion dipped in organic nut butter is very satisfying. Avoid milk chocolate.

SAMPLE MEALS FOLLOWING THESE GUIDELINES

Grill a piece of wild salmon or grass-fed beef. Sauté spinach, mushrooms, and onions in grass-fed butter. Make a salad with organic lettuce, organic cucumber, organic tomatoes, and sprouts. Toss the salad in a small amount of homemade vinaigrette and consider adding a couple of avocado slices. Delicious!

Or, for a quicker meal: Take some non-processed turkey breast and wrap it up in some crispy organic romaine lettuce with avocado and other vegetables.

Finally, if you want to keep it simple, just remember two main points. Minimize processed carbohydrates and refined sugars and balance feeding and fasting.

ADDING HEALTHY CARBOHYDRATES

Please pay close attention to the following statement: the food tables above do not list grains, beans and other legumes, potatoes, or lentils. It omits these foods not because they're unhealthy, but because of their carbohydrate content. The above table is designed for those who are trying to change from a sugar-burning metabolism to a fat-burning metabolism. Therefore, we try to limit overall carbohydrate consumption.

We did list fruits in the tables. Fruits are very good for us, and many of them contain high concentrations of compounds that naturally reduce inflammation. However, when initiating weight loss, fruit consumption should be minimized. Once weight loss is initiated, you can add back fruits and gauge how you respond to the inclusion of them in your diet. Some people can tolerate more carbohydrates, some less. We want you to work towards the broadest diet possible for you that sustains a healthy weight while maximizing nutrient consumption.

Immediately below is a list of healthy carbohydrates that you can add to your nutrition program on the days when you increase your carbohydrate consumption. Always stick with healthy, unprocessed carbohydrates, and avoid refined sugars. Also, do not over consume carbohydrates and grains. Try to limit them to two portions daily and use ½ to 1 cup of whatever carbohydrate you choose. There are plenty of good sources of carbohydrates to choose from. Here is our recommended list:

- Organic sweet potatoes, red potatoes, and organic white potatoes in limited portions

- Beans (try to avoid canned beans)
- Lentils
- Quinoa
- Amaranth
- Spelt
- Organic brown rice
- Whole grain barley
- Couscous
- Freekeh
- Whole rye
- Organic whole oats
- Fruit. When sourced properly, fruits are a source of vitamins, minerals, and fiber. This nutrition program limits your fruit intake while you're trying to lose weight. If you choose to make a smoothie as a meal replacement, then have a small amount of fruit; this shouldn't stall your weight loss as long as it's a small quantity. You can also enjoy fruit on your carbohydrate-loading days. If you're not trying to lose weight, I suggest one to two portions of fruit daily. I especially like berries because they contain antioxidants.

Many of my patients have found healthy substitutes for the textures of bread. They use cauliflower, coconut flours, almond flours, and many other healthy options. Once you experience the energy a healthy diet provides you, it will not take long for you to identify the food sources that are pleasing to you. The list above is not exhaustive.

FOODS THAT MUST BE ORGANICALLY PRODUCED

We want you to eat as much organic produce as you can afford to. Since this can be very expensive, we'll provide a list created by the Environmental Working Group, which studied which fruits and vegetables are most important to eat organically. They labeled this group the "Dirty Dozen Plus." If possible, always purchase the following foods from organic sources:

- Apples
- Celery
- Cherry tomatoes
- Cucumbers
- Grapes
- Hot peppers
- Nectarines
- Peaches
- Potatoes
- Spinach
- Strawberries
- Sweet bell peppers
- Kale/collard greens
- Summer squash

DAIRY

I get a lot of questions about dairy. Some people can tolerate dairy and others can't. You will have to decide for yourself which group you fall into. If you do consume dairy, remember always to purchase your products from healthy sources. Since I personally tolerate dairy very well, I eat real cheeses, whole milk from healthy cows, and whole fat Greek yogurt. There is no evidence that low-fat dairy helps with weight loss. If you choose dairy, choose whole fat. Low-fat dairy has more sugar instead of fat; therefore, it increases insulin which increases fat storage.

PROCESSED FATS AND OILS

We recommend that you always avoid trans fats and that you try to avoid industrialized oils such as vegetable oil, canola oil, cottonseed oil, sunflower oil, safflower oil, refined palm oil, soybean oil, peanut oil, corn oil, and any hydrogenated or partially hydrogenated oils.

CAFFEINE

I recommend *never* consuming sugary sodas or energy drinks. However, tea and coffee have potential health benefits. When used in moderation, caffeine is fine for most people. If you enjoy a cup of coffee or tea in the morning, then it's probably fine for your health. If you're trying to lose weight, I recommend you not use any sweeteners. I recommend you experiment with spices such as cinnamon or vanilla to flavor these beverages. If you must sweeten your coffee or tea then use a small amount of stevia or coconut sugar. If you are not trying to lose weight then consider sweetening these beverages with local honey. Each morning, I enjoy two cups of dark roast coffee with organic whole cream. It tastes great and helps me wake up. I have seen no negative impact on my weight or health from this habit. I do *not* have any caffeine later in the day.

ALCOHOL

If you're trying to lose weight, I recommend avoiding alcohol altogether. Alcoholic beverages are heavy in sugar and calories and will definitely affect your ability to lose weight. As a general rule, it's best to limit your overall alcohol intake. A recent review of the five most harmful habit-forming substances rated alcohol as number one. The overall destructive impact of alcohol on individuals and society is greater than that of heroin or crack cocaine.

The themes of this book are awareness and creating a healthy mind to support a purposeful existence, and alcohol can be damaging to those habits and to our brains generally. Alcohol is certainly dangerous when consumed in excess. It also depletes our self-control and disrupts restorative sleep patterns.

There are many reasons to consider minimizing or even eliminating alcohol from your life. Every one of us should desire to learn how to relax, overcome stress, and enjoy ourselves without having to use this substance, and we should be able to cultivate a sense of joy and peace without needing to drink alcohol.

At the same time, the medical evidence suggests that *moderate* alcohol consumption may provide some health benefits. For women, it is recommended to have no more than one portion daily. Men are recommended not to exceed two portions daily. (Note that a 16-ounce, high-gravity beer counts as two portions.) If you're going to consume alcohol, I recommend limiting it to a minority of days of the week and consuming only according to these guidelines.

TO WHEAT OR NOT TO WHEAT?

Now for the controversial part: To wheat or not to wheat—that is the question. I would recommend that you try to avoid wheat products. I know how hard this is. Many of my patients—and I myself—have a long history of enjoying pastas, breads, and many other foods made from wheat. But I've made it clear in this chapter that our primary focus is how you source your foods, and, unfortunately, that is where the problem lies.

Modern wheat is fundamentally different from ancestral wheat. The DNA of the plant is different and the harvesting process is different. In our modern times, I believe it's far easier to maintain a healthy body weight by avoiding wheat products. If you're going to have some wheat, I recommend that you limit it to one day a week. There are many ways to create the textures and flavors of bread and pastas by using other grains and vegetables.

That said, many of my patients continue to eat foods that contain wheat as part of their nutrition plan, and they are able to maintain a healthy weight and have no detectable medical problems. I suggest you experiment with periods of abstinence from wheat and see how you feel and how your body responds.

I also recommend you do the same thing with corn and soybeans. Most sources of corn and soybeans are mass-produced in a manner that renders them unfit for our bodies. I suggest you reduce your intake of these products.

ELIMINATION DIETS

I am often asked about food allergies or intolerance. There is a basic approach to identifying if a food may be causing issues for you. You eliminate the suspected food for a few weeks, and then you just add it back in a high quantity. This is not a perfect method, but it can sometimes help identify foods your body does not handle well. A functional nutritional expert can help you if you find this simplified method does not provide you the answers you are seeking. The most common foods to potentially cause tolerance issues are corn, peanut, dairy, gluten, eggs, soy, wheat, and processed grains..

IS A HIGH-FAT DIET OKAY?

My preferred nutritional approach for myself, my family, and most of my patients is a diet higher in fat and lower in carbohydrates, as I've outlined in this chapter. There is compelling, emerging evidence that most individuals with type 2 diabetes and metabolic syndrome would benefit from a diet higher in fat and lower in carbohydrates. We're seeing these disease states reverse under this type of nutrition plan.

Yet there is still a lot of controversy about the best diet for patients with metabolic syndrome, diabetes, and cardiovascular disease. As of right now, the American Diabetes Association and the American Heart Association do not recommend higher fat/lower carbohydrate diets. These professional groups believe that high-fat diets may lead to atherosclerotic diseases.

These are evidence-based professional associations, and I respect their opinions. At the same time, much of their evidence comes from populations who consume processed and industrialized fats. I believe that if we studied a group of people following a well-sourced diet higher in fat and lower in carbohydrates, then we would see a lower incidence of cardiovascular diseases, metabolic diseases, and cancer.

As of right now, there is no evidence that diets that are higher in fat and eliminate industrialized oils and sugars cause arterial disease. Atherosclerosis is influenced by many variables, including insulin resistance. Inflammation is a major contributor to atherosclerosis. Diets higher in processed foods trigger insulin resistance and inflammation. Hopefully, in the years to come, our studies will provide clear evidence about the best approach to preventing atherosclerosis. Right now, there is no case to be made for the inclusion of sugars and industrialized vegetable oils in our diets.

Still, I would not recommend that you substitute my advice for the guidance of a treating physician who knows you and your medical conditions. If my guidance is in conflict with what your doctor is recommending, then your doctor's guidance should prevail.

FINDING YOUR RHYTHM IN THE LONG TERM

While the specific guidelines of this chapter will likely be important as you make your initial transition from old habits to new ones, eventually you will develop your own guidelines based on what works for you. Once you've begun to settle into a long-term rhythm of healthy eating, the only foods that you must continue to keep out of your diet are the processed and fake foods full of unhealthy fats and sugars. In all other areas, you should feel free to broaden your diet over time.

The food lists I've provided here are intended as a starting template, not a comprehensive list. If you maintain a diet of lean proteins, healthy fats, abundant produce, and small portions of healthy carbohydrates, you should have no trouble maintaining a healthy body weight and improving your health.

FINAL NOTES

1. **Eat clean:** Minimize all processed foods and refined sugars. Eliminate artificial sweeteners, preservatives, additives, and dyes. Avoid MSG and try to avoid GMOs. Eliminate all industrialized fats and oils and all fake fats. Avoid all meat, milk, eggs, and other food products that come from sick animals. Only consume animal products that are derived from humanely treated, healthy animals.

2. **Drink clean:** Drink lots of pure water. Eliminate sodas, diet sodas, sugary juices, mass-produced sports drinks, energy drinks, and all fake beverages. Stay well-hydrated on pure water. Flavoring water with sliced lemon, lime, or oranges is fine. Coffee, tea, and bone broth are fine.

3. **Lower your carbohydrates, keep protein intake moderate, and increase consumption of healthy fats:**

   - If you're trying to lose weight, reduce carbohydrate consumption. Ketogenic diets are usually less than 50 grams of total carbs daily. Low-carbohydrate diets can range from 50 to 175 grams of carbs daily. Moderate carbohydrate diets range from 175 to 250 grams of carbs daily. Find the amount of carbohydrate reduction that initiates weight loss for you.

More importantly, gauge how you feel. The approach that works for you will feel good to you once you have adapted to it. However, you have to allow the adaptation process to occur. It may feel uncomfortable for a few weeks while your body up-regulates the systems to use fatty acids for fuel.

- Maintain moderate protein intake to 0.5-1.0 gram per kilogram of body weight (to calculate your weight in kg, simply divide your weight in pounds by 2.2). Another way of monitoring protein is to keep it at 20-30 percent of total daily calories.

- Increase your consumption of healthy fats, especially omega-3 fatty acids.

- Increase your consumption of non-starchy vegetables, especially those with high nutrient density as listed in our tables.

- Get plenty of non-grain based fiber, a minimum of 25 grams daily but preferably more.

4. **Eat 2-3 meals daily with no snacking. Extend your overnight fast and consider longer durations of fasting. Do not under-eat on non-fasting days. You must learn to control your hunger and cravings.**

5. **You do not need to reduce your daily calories or measure your portions to be healthy and maintain your weight.** Once your body can use its stored fat as a fuel, and your metabolism is in good working order, you will not need to measure your foods or count calories. Staying on a long-term, calorie-restricted diet will not improve your health or your energy.

6. **Your mindset is the most important contributor to your success:** This chapter is lengthy because of the amount of time I spent discussing a philosophy of nutrition and eating. I have found that pretty much all diets work initially. Finding an eating plan to initiate weight loss is easy. The challenge is to maintain a healthy approach to nutrition over a lifetime. Your mindset, your desire, and your will-power are the most important attributes of long term health. Move, sleep, meditate, source your food well, and enjoy your good health and energy.

STEP INTO THE CONSULTATION ROOM

You've started your new health program with exercises to strengthen your thinking and reduce worrying—but you're not yet entirely clear about how those are going to help you. When you come back into my office a few weeks later, you're eager to focus on the painful symptoms that you're dealing with every day. You're overweight, and your body hurts.

We review the lab tests from your last appointment, which included thyroid testing, cholesterol panel, blood counts, menopausal markers, and vitamin levels. Those tests revealed that you have an impaired fasting glucose, elevated triglycerides, and an early risk of diabetes. None of these require immediate treatment, but they are warning signs of future complications. Your other functions turn up normal. Your overall diagnosis is moderate overweight and diffuse myalgia, which is essentially overall body pain, as well as mild depression and sleep disturbances.

Since you've already gotten started on developing new, healthy habits by strengthening your thinking, it's time to turn to your diet. You note that your diet is very casual in the sense that you eat what's convenient; you frequently eat out at restaurants or grab fast food. You say that, basically, you don't pay too much attention to food.

We circle back to the reason you came in today: you haven't felt good in your body in a long time, and you really want to change that. You just want to feel better.

We start to talk through the importance of nutrition—how the nutrients you eat turn into the energy that powers you through the day, and how poor nutrients will lead not only to a lack of energy but to the pain you perpetually feel in your muscles and joints.

I hand over the nutrition tables from this chapter. I explain that if you start to eat natural, unprocessed foods, you'll feel a big difference in your body. If you truly desire to feel better—and I know that you do—then you have to cut out the processed stuff. I explain that you can start today. You can start *right now*. At the end of our consultation, we agree that you'll check back in several weeks, and I leave you with the following steps for immediate action:

- Drink a glass of water several times a day.
- Try to not eat between meals and maintain a 12 hour period

between your last meal of the day and your first meal the next day.

- Eliminate one unhealthy food from your day today that you would have normally eaten.

- After eliminating that unhealthy food, remind yourself that you're *happy* to give it up, because it's a sign of your success.

- Get to know the attached tables for healthier eating. As soon as you have time, go to the grocery store, food co-op, or natural foods store and begin to source your diet in this new way.

- Before you go to sleep tonight, write down what you ate today. Let those notes become the beginning of a habit journal in which you record your habits from the day and reflect on which ones are moving you toward your goals and which are moving you further away. As much as possible, start tracking everything you're eating and notice what you're feeling before you eat it. Why are you choosing the foods you choose?

ADDITIONAL RESOURCES

- *Deep Nutrition* by Cate Shanahan M.D.

- *In Defense of Food* by Michael Pollan

- Any book by Gary Taubes

- *The Keto Reset Diet* by Mark Sisson and Brad kearns

- *Keto Clarity: Your Definitive Guide to the Benefits of a Low-Carb, High-Fat Diet* by Jimmy Moore with Eric C. Westman, M.D.

- Fitday app or My Fitness pal app for food tracking

- Our resources at healthshepherds.com

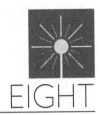

EIGHT

Physical Activity: Play Your Way to Better Health

In this chapter you'll learn how and why physical activity is essential for your metabolism and your health, and you'll find simple guidance for how to incorporate activity into your life in a sustainable way.

IMAGINE FOR A MOMENT that I can write you a prescription for the pill you've been waiting for. You've gone to see your doctor dozens of times because your energy is low and your body hurts, you can't sleep, and you generally don't feel well. Now—finally—the right drug has come on the market. It's going to improve your energy and your focus and your mood. You'll lose weight. You'll sleep well. And your body is going to hurt a whole lot less; maybe it won't hurt at all. On top of that, there are no side effects to this drug as long as it's used as directed. Plus: It's free. Zero co-pay.

My guess is you'd want me to write that prescription immediately.

Of course, there's no pill that can do all of that for you—for some good reasons that I'll explain in a second. But by applying a very simple formula and making a couple of small changes to your life, you can achieve all of those benefits and feel better than you can presently imagine.

You've probably seen plenty of ads on TV for exercise machines that are supposedly all-in-one fitness solutions. You've probably heard of the craze for CrossFit and Zumba and other programs. Maybe along the way you've tried a few of them. And maybe you quickly found that they were too time-consuming or too expensive or too painful. I have nothing against those programs. If you find they work well for you, then I think that is great. However, rest assured: this chapter is not going to ask you to commit to one specific program.

The solution that you'll find in these pages promises similar results to all of those exercise fads—but it's free, it doesn't take much time, and it's sustainable. That is, it's not designed to sell you a product, but rather to get you started on a regimen that's simple and easy enough to incorporate into your life in perpetuity. It's not a fad that you'll do three days a week for two months and then never do again.

By this point in the book, you also know that your health is largely the result of your habits. *Everything* is a habit: how you sit, stand, walk, breathe, and whether you choose to exercise. Your overall biomechanical health—that is, the actual physical machine of your body, how it works, whether it can do what you ask of it, and whether it's in pain—is primarily a product of habit, too. This book is all about converting your existing habits into ones that will make you biomechanically healthy.

The first and most powerful of all your habits is your thinking, as we talked about in Chapter Four. So take a moment right now to call to mind the goals you've set for yourself. Focus on a very clear picture of the healthy version of yourself that you're moving toward. Regardless of where you are today, regardless of the ailments that have restricted your life up until now, know that if you apply the simple guidelines in this chapter, you will be capable of turning into that healthy version of yourself. Then you'll have more physical and emotional and mental energy to put toward your purpose in life.

We're now going to turn to a formula that's every bit as powerful as that magic prescription pill. This formula has five basic parts to it:

- Biomechanical awareness: Become aware of what's happening within your body.

- Postural awareness: Become aware of how you're holding your body.

- Activity: Start moving your body.

- Strength: Maintain your lean body mass.

- Rest: Give your body generous time to rest and recover.

THE OVERALL POINT IS *MOVEMENT*: MOVEMENT BEGETS LIFE

More than anything else, I want you to move. Take every opportunity to walk, stretch, squat, lift, pull, push, hang, and any other thing that makes use of the physical machine known as your body. Your body is designed for movement, for physical engagement.

I want your physical body to become a source of pleasure for you. I want you to move your body and rest your body in a manner consistent with its design. Our modern environments have been so heavily engineered to be comfortable that they are basically unnatural. Your body is designed to heat itself and cool itself. It is designed to adapt to different environments. Your body is designed for many types of movement. Maintaining a sitting position most of the time causes biomechanical diseases. Physical inactivity sends the wrong messages to your physiology.

We are designed for movement, not sitting. Just like we need to balance fasting and feeding, we need to balance physical activity and resting. Just like eating too frequently influences obesity and metabolic diseases, physical inactivity influences biomechanical diseases. This is the same principle that runs through this entire book. We must use our body and mind as designed. Your body is designed for movement.

AWARENESS OF WHAT'S HAPPENING WITHIN YOUR BODY

Many patients come into my office with biomechanical problems. Their bodies are breaking down in a way that's causing them discomfort; they can't do the activities they used to do or they're experiencing regular pain or stiffness. They also tend to feel tired a lot of the time. And all of that affects their quality of life and their ability to function on a daily basis, both at work and in their leisure activities.

Historically, the way the medical field has dealt with this type of biomechanical problem was with X-rays and diagnoses that included arthritis, tendinitis, bursitis, and muscular strain. The doctor would write a prescription for an anti-inflammatory medication, plus maybe a muscle relaxer or a pain pill, and the patient was told to come back if he or she didn't get better. Occasionally physical therapy was also considered as an option, though it was typically a type of physical therapy that was expensive and involved frequent and time-consuming visits to a trainer. Not surprisingly, that old formula hasn't solved our problems.

This book's approach to biomechanical health is very different. It starts by focusing on the fact that your biomechanical system is your body's connective tissue; it's what holds you up against gravity, and it's what allows you to move.

Much of modern life—such as our forms of entertainment, our typically sedentary jobs, and the positions we sit in—tends to be detrimental to our biomechanics. Very often, by the time we feel the pain that comes from enduring so many unhealthy circumstances, we've already done quite a bit of damage. We might even have started compensating for that damage with unconscious physical habits that create still more damage and pain. That's why awareness is the very first step on this path toward improved physical health.

So, for starters, I'm asking you to focus on how you're engaging your body throughout the day, whether you're at work or relaxing. Just try to notice and feel the different muscles and body parts that you're using and how they engage. Feel your shoulders and the muscles of your torso engage as you lift, bend, twist, turn, and move through all your different activities. And if you have an area of significant or consistent discomfort, start to really notice where and when it hurts.

This simple awareness is going to have some important results. The process of becoming aware of your body and the positions you find yourself in—and paying attention to your muscles, their function, and how they feel—will actually help you protect your biomechanical health.

I know that this might sound like a lot of work at first. You might be wondering how you can possibly pay attention to everything going on in your body while you have so many other responsibilities throughout the day. Well, at the very beginning, this *will* take some focus and mental energy—that's true. But it all goes back to habit. Eventually, this type of awareness will become your habit, and at that point it won't take mental energy from you. On the contrary, really putting your focus on your body, on your biomechanical structure and how it's engaging throughout the day, will give you clarity. It will make you feel stronger and more confident. It will lift you up emotionally.

AWARENESS OF HOW YOU'RE HOLDING YOUR BODY

The next step is to key in to your posture. Whether you're sitting or lying down or standing at this moment as you read (or listen to) this book, consider whether you're holding your head straight up and back—or is it, instead, drooped forward? Are your shoulders rolled forward and slumped, or are they held back in a dignified position? Is your body tense? Is your jaw clenched? Do you feel tension in your head, perhaps the beginning of a tension headache? How does it feel in your back and in your core at this moment? How does it feel in your legs? Do you feel pain or fatigue? Does your body feel like it's supporting you in the activity of reading this book at this moment, or does it feel instead as if it's being drained of energy?

Now take a moment to straighten your back, to tighten your tummy, to bring your shoulders into a rolled back and open position, to lift your neck up and your chin back in order to get yourself into a good, erect posture. Once you've done that, notice if you don't already feel a little different, a little more tuned in to what's really happening in your body, and maybe even a little more confident.

Most of the people who come into my office are slumped over. Their shoulders are rolled forward. They're tight, and they're in pain. The relatively simple act of taking inventory of their body and correcting their posture can go a long way toward lessening the pain they feel on a regular basis. That's why awareness—first of your biomechanics, and now of your posture—is so central to this formula for improving physical well-being.

Below are detailed pictures of the right way to hold your body when you're standing. Take a look at the image of someone with good posture as compared to bad posture. Look at the position of her head relative to her shoulders, look at how her shoulders are rolled down and back away from her ears. Try to mimic that for yourself. See what it feels like. Consider having someone else watch you as you do this, and then have that person compare your posture to the picture. That will help you see what you can't see for yourself.

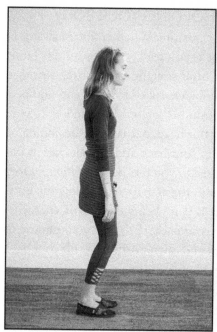 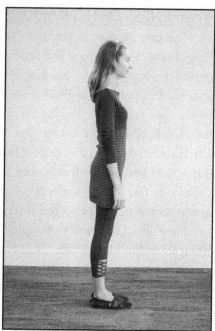

Bad posture   Good posture

For additional, detailed pictures on sitting and standing as well as on walking, bending, and lifting, please refer to our online resource at www. healthshepherds.com.

When you get yourself into the right position, you'll feel that your belly is firmer but not under pressure, your back feels solidly engaged in supporting your torso, your shoulders feel free and energized for action, and that the crown of your head is lifted. Though it may seem hard to believe right now, turning this healthy posture into a habit will be power-ful enough, all by itself, to reduce a host of problems—everything from headaches to neck and back pain to excruciating muscle spasms to nerve entrapment in your arms.

At first, it will be tricky to maintain a healthy posture, though. You'll take inventory and correct yourself—and then a couple of minutes later, your body will resume its usual, slumped position. That's because the old position is a habit, and developing new habits takes time.

But by taking inventory of your body position several times through-out the day and persistently correcting yourself, you'll eventually settle into a new habit. Your body will begin to remember to maintain the healthy position. Start by simply taking inventory of your body, pulling yourself into a healthy posture, and then repeating that as often as you can.

Tai-chi is an excellent, structured discipline to help improve your biomechanical awareness. Consider working with a kinesiology professional to improve this essential skill. I also strongly recommend exploring Katie Bowman's work, which is available at nutritiousmovement.com. She has a great learning platform on which to rebuild your biomechanical health.

You might also need to make a few tweaks to your physical environment. "Ergonomics" is the study of how your environment is suited to your body. And though it's usually not too difficult to change your environment so that it facilitates good posture and helps you avoid injury, it does require that you do an assessment and then make any necessary modifications.

If you work at a desk and you're slouched over all day, you're going to have problems. Eventually you'll have pain and dysfunction, and you'll need medication or surgery. So the way you set up your workstation is very important. You've got to arrange it so that you're sitting with your shoulders and head in the right position.

Happily, we're now at the point where most employers recognize the importance of this issue, and there may be support at your job to help you. Some places offer special chairs that give the right kind of lumbar support. Other offices encourage employees to sit on a stability ball. Still others offer standing or elevated desks. And even if your employer doesn't have any of these resources, you can use the pictures in this book and in our online resource to identify anything in your current setup that's forcing your body into a bad posture. Then you can do things as simple as using old phone books to raise the height of your computer monitor, or changing the height of your chair and adjusting the placement of your keyboard.

If you don't work at a desk, it will be important for you to use the included resources to pay close attention to your standing posture, as well as to your posture as you bend over and lift objects, if that's part of your work.

Also take the time to ensure that your car seat and your bed and your home are all facilitating a healthy body position. That may mean buying a few special pillows or trading out an old chair or simply paying attention to the way you lie down to rest at night.

If you find yourself tempted to skip all this, or if you begin to feel that regularly correcting your posture is tiresome, just remember: this is the route to the good health you want for yourself!

START MOVING—AND *PLAYING*

The next step on your road to biomechanical health is even more straightforward than the first two. It's as simple as moving your body for at least a few minutes a day. If that doesn't sound simple and instead feels daunting, don't worry. I'm going to explain how you can turn physical activity into an enjoyable habit that doesn't seem difficult or burdensome— even as it delivers extraordinary health benefits.

The truth is that, over the past sixty years or so, we've taken our environment and engineered it primarily for comfort. We sit in our cars, we sit at our desks, and we sit in our chairs at home. But the sitting position, in which we now spend practically all of our waking hours, is not at all consistent with how the human body has been used throughout history. We've gotten to the point now where we resist just about all types of movement. We take the elevator; we don't even want to bend over to pick something up off the floor.

But movement is health. If, instead of arranging our physical environment to minimize movement, we set up our environment for *maximum* movement—including reaching and bending and walking and stretching and moving around, all day long, just as we have throughout human existence—we would begin to feel entirely different in our bodies. We wouldn't have to set aside specific time for exercise, because our daily lives would be exercising our bodies. And that, by itself, would go a long way toward keeping us well.

Epigenetics has something to say about the topic of exercise, too. Movement directly affects how your DNA expresses itself. The more we move, the more we up-regulate our metabolism. People who move more will have more muscle mass, because that's how the body's DNA is expressing itself. The individual cells in our bodies respond to the pressures they encounter as we move through our environment—including the pressures of movement and exercise—and those pressures actually change how your cells express themselves. Movement will optimize your genetic expression for physical vitality.

Indeed, the evidence on the health benefits of physical activity is astounding. Back in Chapter Two, I described how I went on something of a journey to find the best comprehensive guidance for my many patients who were coming in with complicated health problems that couldn't be solved with a prescription drug. Well, one of the major things I discovered is that the health statistics for people who are physically active are wildly different from those who are inactive. Inactive people have a higher incidence of just about every possible ailment, from obesity and diabetes and high blood pressure to high cholesterol, arterial disease, certain cancers, sleep apnea, chronic digestive issues, anxiety, depression, and many other problems.

In other words, we *know* that inactivity will cause disease. And here's the reason that there's no magic pill that can solve this problem in the way I described at the beginning of the chapter: we have to use our bodies in accordance with the way they were designed, and you can't do that with a pill.

Just as we need air in our lungs and we need to drink when we're thirsty, physical activity is no different; it's an essential function. Our bodies were designed for activity and mobility. If we don't use them that way, they'll break down. They'll begin to suffer joint pain, muscle pain, and spinal disease. All of that pain will cause depression, fatigue, and stress, and each of those things will create additional negative cycles. Over long periods of time, inactivity can lead to debility and permanent loss of function. Ultimately, the lesson is straightforward: in order to feel good, we have to move our bodies.

You may have been hearing this same advice—that you should exercise—for most of your life. Right now, you may be wondering how my recommendation is any different. Well, strange as it may sound, I can relate.

Since I was a kid, I was always told that I should exercise. I was told it was something I *had* to do. And that made me not want to do it. Even though there were sports that I really enjoyed playing, I didn't consider those "exercise." To me, exercise was *work*—something that I didn't want to do but that I was always *supposed* to do.

Yet I was happy to play baseball with my friends all day long. That wasn't work; it was *purpose*. It was the purpose I felt in doing what I most wanted to do.

So once again, the philosophy of this book comes around to your life's purpose and to what you envision for yourself. I'm going to show you how the physical activity that's going to heal your body *isn't* work; it can be just about any activity you enjoy. But we'll get to that in a second.

PUTTING ONE FOOT IN FRONT OF THE OTHER

For all of us who've seen a late-night infomercial for a supposedly "magic" exercise machine that can be yours for "only" twelve easy payments of $19.99, the following piece of evidence-based health advice is nearly priceless: all you really need to do is *walk*.

Walking uses your muscles and your aerobic capacity. It burns calories and it helps you to feel better in both body and mind. If you're physically able to go for walks, walking could be your entire exercise program. That would do the trick. (If you're unable to walk, don't worry. You have options. I'll discuss them shortly.)

Walking outside is especially beneficial. The act of getting outdoors and into the sunlight and engaging with the environment has benefits over and above the physical act of walking. Seeing some trees and shrubs and potentially a few flowers and birds will help you to feel more tuned in to the world around you and more a part of something greater. It can give you mental clarity.

Yet if for any reason you're unable to walk outside, then walk inside. Walk up the steps. Walk around your office. Walk at lunchtime. Walk indoors on a treadmill if you have to. Get up and walk in place if nothing else. But at least get up and walk, because the benefits are profound.

Many communities also have walking groups to provide companionship and motivation for exercise. Perhaps that's the perfect thing for you. Other people would prefer to walk alone; it all depends on what you most enjoy and what will keep you motivated.

It's also important to apply what we talked about in the first half of this chapter to your walking. Tune in to your posture and then correct your body position using the pictures provided in our online resources. Notice which muscles you're using and how your body feels. Create a method of walking in which you're engaging your core and your abdominal and back muscles.

Sometimes, if we're not thinking about it, we actually walk in a way that creates stress. When you walk correctly, there won't be any unnecessary impact on your knees and feet or pain in your back. Walking with correct posture will also naturally strengthen your muscles. Again, refer to our electronic resource to make sure you've got your body in the right position, and see if a family member or friend will take a look at the pictures and at your posture in order to help you.

Once you've begun to develop a habit of walking, there are a few things to incorporate to create additional health benefits. If you're walking outdoors, walk uphill. And while you're walking uphill, try to walk just as quickly as you normally do, so that you start to breathe harder. If you're indoors on a treadmill, use the incline function or increase the pace. It's important to enjoy yourself while you're walking—but it's also good to push yourself periodically. You should experience some shortness of breath and an increase in your heart rate, because that will improve your physical conditioning and make you healthier.

Walking and running are great, but these activities do tighten up your hips and hamstrings. Frequently, I see patients who are really enjoying a walking-based movement program but then start to develop hip bursitis and something known as IT band syndrome. These ailments can be prevented by stretching the hips and hamstrings regularly. Foam rolling and massages (especially something known as vacuum therapy) are great interventions to keep the hips and hamstrings healthy. Walk as much as you are able to, but also take time for stretching and myofascial release (muscle relaxing). Do not wait until you have pain to start the supportive activities that will keep you moving.

If walking isn't possible for you, that's not a reason to worry. You have options. The goal is simply to get your body moving. Can you get into the swimming pool at the local YMCA? Can you use a stationary bike? An elliptical machine? A rowing machine? Can you find something else—just about anything else, really—that gets you moving?

And whether you can walk or not, consider simply going out to *play*. Play golf, play tennis, go to the park, roll around with your kids. Play whiffle ball, badminton, softball, volleyball, or go swimming. Work in your garden. Take some time to think about which physical activities you most enjoy—or which ones you *used* to enjoy, before your body started to hurt the way it does now. Maybe you can't play softball just yet—but maybe once you start walking regularly, you'll be able to.

I know a guy who retired to Florida, and you know what his favorite retirement activity is? Softball! He plays in the local league year-round. Of course, you might not like softball one bit—and that's fine. You might want to organize your bookshelves and then plant geraniums by your front door. You should do whichever activities feel playful to you, and do them outdoors as much as possible. Experiment! Try new things as well as old things that you used to love. Just go *play*!

Most of all, the key is to find activities that feel joyful and fulfilling. That will keep both your mind and body engaged and healthy. It will keep your brain growing and your physical machine working. It will facilitate mental clarity, a sense of purpose, and emotional resiliency. And eventually, over time, you won't have to think about being active—because it will have become a habit. As Nike says, you'll *just do it*.

And the more you do it, the more others around you will want to be part of it. Because when you're having fun and feeling joyful, that's attractive to others. You'll become a source of positivity and well-being for those around you, which will help influence your friends and family to find their way back to good health, too.

HOW MUCH IS ENOUGH?

If you become physically active doing things that feel like play instead of work, you probably won't have to worry about getting *enough* activity—because when something is fun, you tend to do it as much as you can. But of course, that's not your starting point. At first, and for a little while, physical activity might feel onerous and uncomfortable. That's completely natural. That leads many people to ask, "Doc, how much time do I really *have* to spend being physically active?"

It's a good question, because there's a lot of confusion out there. Some studies say you need to exercise forty-five minutes a day, six days a week. Other studies say you don't need that much in order to be healthy. So which is it?

The answer is simple: just do what you can. No amount of time is too short. If all you can spare is five minutes, then get up and walk for five minutes. If you can walk for an hour and you feel good, then go for an hour. Do whatever you can. And any time it starts to feel like too much, take a break. Rest. Breathe. Drink fluids. Then start again. (Rest, in fact, is the last part of our formula for good biomechanical health; I'll say more about it momentarily.)

If you do all of that—and if you really put your effort into it and pay attention to your posture while you're doing it—then ultimately, you're going to succeed.

It's extremely important that your exercise not become yet another onerous responsibility in your life. That's why I'm emphasizing the playful aspect of it. You don't want to get into a mindset where you feel guilty because you "skipped" your obligatory exercise. That guilt may make you even *less* likely, rather than more likely, to exercise the next day, or the next. You just want to focus on making movement a *habit*.

Developing an movement habit will take time, in the same way that it will take time for you to make good posture a habit. And just as with your posture, when you realize that you haven't moved your body in a while, just get out there and do it. If all you have is five minutes, then take those five minutes. Maybe you'll have an hour on the weekend. Move your body to whatever extent you're able. Just make it a habit!

MAINTAINING YOUR LEAN BODY MASS

The concept of "lean body mass" is essentially how much muscle you have on your body. It's an important topic because a decline in lean body mass—through inactivity or the natural aging process—brings with it some serious negative effects. Less lean body mass means a lower metabolism and an increased likelihood of weight gain. It also triggers a decline in hormone production, loss of bone density, and greater risk of metabolic disease. People who maintain their lean body mass not only have better bone density, better hormonal function, and a lower body fat percentage, but they also report a greater sense of well-being.

That raises an obvious question: *how* do you maintain lean body mass? It's actually pretty simple—you just have to use your muscles. When you use them, they strengthen and grow. When you don't use them, they atrophy.

If you're someone who hasn't been using your muscles for a while, then your muscle fibers are basically "sleeping." What we're going to do is wake them up and recruit them into activity. Some people will see rapid results from doing this—they'll feel sore, but they'll experience a quick improvement in strength, which can be really gratifying. For other people this process will be harder. Some people will have actually lost muscle fiber through inactivity, and thus they'll need not only to wake up the fibers but to rebuild them as well. That takes more time, but the process isn't complicated.

In either case, we're going to use a program of resistance training in order to maintain and build your lean body mass. "Resistance training" just means putting your muscles under a certain amount of tension and briefly holding that tension. That actually sends a message to each muscle to increase its own capacity by recruiting more muscle fibers—or, simply put, it tells the muscle to grow.

We've created an online resource for this program, which you can access at www.healthshepherds.com. Our program is a set of short and efficient resistance-training exercises in a style that's known as "high-intensity interval training," or HIIT. In our electronic resource, you'll find a sequence of five exercises that use the resistance of your own body weight to build muscle (and for those of you who are more advanced, you can opt to use stretch bands or free weights as well). We perform each exercise for forty-five seconds in a direct sequence, and then repeat it four times, which adds up to a total of fifteen minutes. We recommend doing this fifteen-minute sequence three times a week. (Note that you don't have to use our specific HIIT program; there are many resistance-training resources out there, and you should feel free to use whichever one suits you best.)

If you use our program, it will not take you long to figure out that it's a pretty simple formula. Essentially, we are suggesting you use a sequence of a pull, a press, a squat, a lunge, and one other type of motion to place all of your major muscle groups under stress. That stress will initiate a reparative hormonal response that will improve your overall health.

You can choose from hundreds of different motions using body weight, free weights, or stretch bands and create your own program over time. The key is to focus on form and the full and sustained contraction of all your muscles to achieve the desired response from your body. Go slowly and focus on sustained muscle contractions rather than counting reps and trying to achieve a certain number. It's about the *effort*, not the quantity.

You could even do a ten-minute version of this in your business clothes on a short break during your workday. If you do not have time to go to the gym, it doesn't matter. Just pick a sequence of exercises and rotate through them continuously for five, ten, or fifteen minutes. You could do three lower-body exercises in ten minutes on one day, and then three upper-body exercises in ten minutes the next day, and continue to alternate days. No matter your age, your physical limitations, your time, or your access to a workout facility, you will always have an effective way of maintaining a vitalized, lean body mass.

This fifteen-minute program will send your body all the right physiological cues that are necessary for increasing your lean body mass. And this program is designed to work for *every*body, whether you're 25 and a former athlete or you're 70 years old and simply trying to build or rebuild good health.

It's important that you maintain the same biomechanical awareness that we discussed at the beginning of this chapter while you go through these exercises. Focus on engaging each muscle. Minimize any weights that you may be using. Don't worry about how many repetitions you're doing. In fact, if you do these exercises with no additional weight whatsoever and go very slowly, completely focused on form, I assure you that you will have done everything necessary to see results.

The effects of doing this type of exercise can be tremendous. By engaging in this program, you'll increase your resting metabolic rate, burn calories, reduce insulin resistance and the risk of diabetes, lower your blood pressure, improve your ability to sleep soundly at night, and release endorphins to create a greater sense of well-being.

Engaging in some form of exercise that puts your muscles under stress to the point of failure, regardless of your age or conditioning status, is imperative for your overall health. Without it, you aren't tapping into a major resource for feeling your best and for unlocking your body's potential to use fat metabolically as fuel, and to build muscle and repair tissue.

If you'd like to go even further to build your lean body mass, I recommend yoga, Pilates, plyometrics, or heavier lifting routines (with a trainer, preferably). One of the great things about all of these forms of exercise is that they emphasize breathing and remaining focused during the stress of challenging poses. That brings with it tremendous side benefits, including reducing anxiety and sharpening mental clarity. At the same time, you'll improve core muscle strength, overall muscle tone, and mobility of your joints. That's a pretty great payoff.

I personally like to be outdoors as much as possible. I take lots of walks with my dog and my family. I have always enjoyed running and try to keep up a running habit. Sometimes I run at a gentle pace and just focus on my breathing. It becomes a form of meditation for me that is very relaxing.

Sometimes I will integrate different forms of sprints into my runs. I may use a series of all-out ten second sprints interspersed with periods of light jogging or walking. I will sometimes do moderate distance sprints of 200-400 yards. Sometimes I skip or run backwards for a bit. The reason for all of this variation is I am trying to stimulate all of my body's energy systems. We have many different energy pathways in the body, and these different types of sprinting activate the different pathways. This improves metabolic function. This can be done with any type of endurance activity.

I find tabata training quite effective when time is limited. Pick a movement such as a burpee and do it for twenty seconds followed by ten seconds of rest. Repeat this eight times for a very effective four minute workout. There are many examples of tabata movements available on the internet. Strengthening your body does not have to take a lot of time.

I also try to sneak in push-ups, pull-ups, planks, squats, and lunges throughout my day. I just want my muscles and joints to feel stimulated. In between patient visits, I will sometimes just close the exam room door and do push-ups or squats. I am sure my team members will get a chuckle when they read this, and picture me, a middle aged man in khakis and a button down shirt, doing push-ups in an exam room.

One last thing about this. It is perfectly fine to initiate physical activity while fasting. You do not have to eat to exercise. Your body has plenty of stored energy to use for physical activity. In fact, as we discussed earlier, fasting upregulates growth hormone and sympathetic nervous system hormones so it may be an optimal time for exercise. Do not feel you have to eat in order to engage in physical activity. Exercise can actually turn your hunger off.

ALLOW YOUR BODY TO REST AND RECOVER

It's absolutely *essential* that you let your body rest from exercise. Many of us feel an urgency to achieve quick results, and sometimes that means we don't rest, even when our bodies are telling us to do so. But pushing ahead instead of resting *won't* help you achieve quicker results. On the contrary, the *more* you rest during this type of activity, the *faster* you'll get where you want to go, because rest allows your body to rebuild.

Adding a resting phase is consistent with our overall philosophy in this book. This is about building and maintaining lifelong health—not having a flatter tummy in six weeks. So take your time. Become aware and maintain that awareness as you work your way through these programs. Take plenty of rest and recovery breaks along the way.

Rest is vital because of the way your body responds to exercise. When you take your muscles to their limits—that is, to their physiological threshold of failure—your body will react. During the course of your workout, you'll likely feel short of breath. You might start to feel heavy, or you'll have a feeling of warmth or swollenness or soreness in your muscles. All of those are indications that you pushed your muscles to the right threshold.

Then your body will have a hormonal response. For up to forty-eight hours after you stress your muscles, your metabolism will be faster. That's because you secrete cortisol and catecholamines during your workouts, and those are hormones that release both fat and sugar into your bloodstream to be burned as fuel.

Through working your body, you begin to tap into your body's ability to burn fat, which helps reduce your insulin resistance. The effect lasts for up to forty-eight hours after working out, so you want to be sure to give yourself time to cycle through those responses.

But the second lesson is to take all the rest you need between these workouts. You may choose to do your lean-body-mass exercises once, twice, or three times a week—but don't do them every day. Give yourself a minimum of forty-eight hours in between workouts. Doing the exercises every day won't help you achieve your goals. In fact, there are a number of good scientific studies that show that even one 15-minute strength workout per week, in which you take all of your muscles to the threshold of failure, is all you need to maintain your lean body mass. Furthermore, research indicates that the more rest you get, the more likely you'll get stronger.

Your rest and recovery process can include a number of different things. It could be just basic physical rest. It could also mean working with a physical therapist, where you do stretches, self-massage, a technique called myofascial release, or foam rolling to improve the mobility of your joints, reduce adhesions in your connective tissue, and reduce muscle pain and tightness.

I would also strongly recommend working with an integrative biomechanical expert who knows you. This person might be a medical manual therapist (sometimes referred to as a massage therapist), chiropractor, physical therapist, acupuncturist, or an exercise physiologist. What these experts do is very important for overall health. They are able to lengthen muscles and reduce trigger points in your body, and they can help reduce chronic strain.

Medical manual therapy, chiropractic adjustments, physical therapy, yoga, meditation and controlled breathing, and getting good sleep each night are all ways of allowing your body to rest and recover. They keep your body in balance, optimize your physical health, and reduce your chance of injury.

However you decide to structure your rest and recovery time, the bottom line is clear: rest is a crucial part of biomechanical health.

Let me emphasize once more the basic concept of movement: I just want you to *move*. Set up your environment so you can maximize your movement. Keep foam rollers and massage balls around your home and your workplace, and put them to use frequently. While you're talking with your family in the evening, roll your feet on a small ball and stretch your toes. Try to maximize your movement and continuously explore new ways of using your body.

Embrace the idea of picking things up, taking two trips up the stairs, squatting down, and any other movement. I also strongly recommend you visit nutritiousmovement.com and explore the excellent resources on movement and physical health that Katie Bowman has put together.

STEP INTO THE CONSULTATION ROOM

When you come back to my office, you report that you've started to feel a little better, thanks to the changes in your diet. That's great news! And now we turn our focus to another, and equally important, driver of your health.

"How physically active are you?" I ask.

You explain that, although you try to exercise, you're so busy that it rarely happens.

I ask about your job and whether you're active or sedentary throughout the day. You explain that your job involves sitting at a computer. You have started to walk 15 minutes a day. When I ask, you say that you otherwise haven't given much thought to your posture or physical movement. Your employer has never provided an ergonomic assessment of your workstation.

We return to the notion of habit. Since our last appointment, you've been keeping a daily inventory of some of your habits. I suggest that you expand that journaling and track how you're feeling at different points throughout the day. Are you stressed or calm, tired or energetic? The idea is to start to pay attention to which circumstances lead to which emotional states.

You're also going to keep track of your physical activity. How often are you moving your body? Then do the same for your biomechanics—how are you sitting? Is your back straight, or slumped? Do your desk and chair actually fit your body? How are you breathing? Are you taking short, shallow breaths, or deep breaths that help you relax?

Taking inventory in this way is a powerful next step on your path toward health. As you begin to become aware of your habits, you'll have greater insight into what makes you feel healthy and what makes you feel sick. At the end of the consultation, we settle on the following plan:

- You resolve to stop and simply notice your body position three times a day. If you notice that you're slouched, you'll take a second to straighten yourself into an upright and dignified position.

- You agree to do a 15- to 30-minute biomechanical awareness program twice weekly. That means yoga, tai chi, Pilates, or using a foam roller on sore muscle groups.

- You commit to 15 to 30 minutes of brisk walking three to five days a week.

- I print off a set of strengthening exercises, and you decide that you'll do them at least once a week.

- You agree that, as you get used to this program of taking inventory of your habits, becoming active, and striving to maintain better body position, you'll also consider adding some new activities. You recall that you used to enjoy playing kick ball. You decide that you'd like to get yourself into good enough shape to be able to do that with your kids. You also like the idea of taking up gardening.

You leave the appointment feeling optimistic—and surprised. For a long time, you've thought that exercise was difficult and painful. But the walking you've been doing since your first appointment several weeks ago actually has you feeling pretty good. Doing strength exercises once a week seems like it will not be too burdensome. You decide that you'll be outside playing with your kids in no time.

Actually, this is the first time you've ever thought about your total daily movement as *exercise*. You're no longer worrying about how you're going to find time for exercise, because finding spare time for a new activity always felt difficult or even impossible. You see now that movement is a part your daily routine, and you're simply looking for ways to make it an even bigger part of your day. That doesn't feel like work. Suddenly, you *want* to move.

ADDITIONAL RESOURCES

- "Nutritious Movement: You Are How You Move" at www. nutritiousmovement.com

- *You Are Your Own Gym: The Bible of Bodyweight Exercises* by Mark Lauren and Joshua Clark

- *True to Form* by Dr. Eric Goodman (I strongly recommend this book)

- Our resources at www.healthshepherds.com

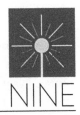

NINE

Why You Need to Sleep More, and Sleep Better

In this chapter you'll learn why sleep is absolutely essential to your health and why both quality and quantity of sleep matter, and you'll find simple guidelines to help you become an expert sleeper.

"I'M JUST EXHAUSTED all the time."

Ryan sat in an exam room in my office, one shirt sleeve rolled up from having his blood pressure taken, and he was unhappy. Ryan had been to my office a number of times to see me about fatigue. He also struggled with generalized pain in his body, and he was overweight.

"There's got to be something going on," he said, shaking his head. "I did some reading on this, and I'm wondering if maybe I have a thyroid problem?"

So we ran the appropriate tests. We checked his hormone levels, his thyroid, and his blood sugar. We checked his blood count to make sure he wasn't anemic. But all the tests came back normal.

I asked him how he was sleeping at night.

"Sometimes I'm restless, I guess," he said. "And I snore. But I don't think that's the problem. There has to be something bigger than that."

I suggested a home screening, in which Ryan would wear a device as he slept in order to measure his oxygen intake and heart rate. That way, we would find out if he was breathing adequately at night and, more generally, if he was getting the sort of restful, restorative sleep that's necessary for good health.

And what did we find?

We discovered that Ryan was getting practically no restorative sleep at all. In fact, he was significantly under-breathing throughout the night, meaning his body was actually *stressing out* while he slept. He was enduring more physical stress at night than he was during the day. Not surprisingly, this lack of healthy sleep had been causing a bunch of health problems including inflammation, mental and physical fatigue, continued weight gain, and some early signs of insulin resistance. When Ryan heard all that, he was eager to do whatever he could to start sleeping well at night. So we began working together to get him into a healthy routine. And as soon as he started getting restorative sleep, he began to feel different. He had energy. He wasn't in pain. And that was the beginning of a transformation in which Ryan also lost weight and became healthier than he'd been in years.

Ryan isn't a special case. In fact, sleep issues are one of the top reasons people go to the doctor. At the same time, far too many of us underestimate the importance of good sleep.

In the last chapter I explained that physical activity is essential because of the way our bodies are designed; there's just no substitute for moving our bodies, because our bodies were made to move. Sleep is the same. In just the way that you have to move your body and breathe air into your lungs and drink when you're thirsty, you've got to sleep. If you're not getting adequate rest, then the health of your mind and body will be compromised.

But there's good news. For the vast majority of people, it's pretty easy to make the right changes in order to get the restorative sleep they need.

And as with each topic we've dealt with in this book, making those changes begins with your thinking. Right now, you might be someone who doesn't prioritize sleep; you might have always considered it unimportant. Now is the time to change that mindset and to cultivate a genuine *desire* for sleep.

With that desire as your motivation, we'll then turn to your habits. This chapter will allow you to assess which of your habits are keeping you from sleeping well, and you'll learn how to change those habits for the better. But before we get to that, you'll find important information about why your body requires restorative sleep. Having this information will help you take better care of yourself.

HOW SLEEP MAKES YOU HEALTHY—
AND HOW A LACK OF SLEEP MAKES YOU SICK

Why is sleep so vitally important?

Consider the fact that your body goes through certain physiological processes by which it repairs and restores itself. Your daily activity—no matter what it is—inflicts wear and tear on you in body and mind. Then your body and brain automatically repair that damage through basic physiological processes—while you sleep. If you're not getting deep sleep, or if you're not getting enough of it, you'll start to suffer.

To picture what I mean by this, think of your brain activity as a process similar to making dinner for your family. You fix a nice meal and get it on the table, but food waste accumulates as you do so. Maybe it's broccoli stems and chicken bones, or maybe it's eggshells when you're making omelets. Whatever's on the menu, there's always some waste. Now imagine if you never cleared away that waste; imagine if you *never* took out the trash. Then picture trying to cook dinner for your family in a kitchen that's crowded with months'—or years'—worth of garbage. Surrounded by that mess, you'd have to work harder and harder just to make a simple dinner for your family.

That's more or less what you're doing to yourself when you don't sleep. You're accumulating waste products in a way that prevents you from functioning normally. The synapses in your brain can't work as they're supposed to because they're drowning in waste; a sustained lack of sleep will erode your ability to think and focus as well as to learn new things and remember them. Your adrenal gland function and your sympathetic nervous system will go into overdrive. You'll experience fatigue and inflammation.

Study after study has demonstrated how much our mental performance and focus are affected by sleep deprivation. Studies conducted on military personnel, doctors, and pilots, plus people in other professions, clearly demonstrate that insufficient sleep affects overall productivity as well as mental acuity and memory.

The lack of sleep also affects your overall metabolism and energy. It elevates your heart rate and blood pressure. Insufficient sleep increased blood sugar and insulin resistance. Insufficient sleep raises cortisol levels which is your stress hormone. Your mitochondria are the energy factories of your cells. They produce your energy. When they are not working well, you will have brain fog and fatigue. Insufficient sleep interferes with the function of your mitochondria.

Sleep deprivation can make you gain weight in other ways, too. Insufficient sleep impacts your satiety signaling causing you to eat more. Also, your willpower is reduced and you are more likely to indulge in habits that are not helping you. Insufficient sleep contributes to obesity through a number of pathways. Many individuals will wake at night and then actually get up to have a sugary snack. So you can see how inadequate sleep can be directly related to obesity and, in some cases, to diabetes as well.

Sleep deprivation also increases the likelihood that you'll suffer from a host of other conditions. It brings an increased risk of cardiovascular problems and coronary artery disease. It can lead to anxiety and depression. It increases the chances that you'll have migraines. And, as if all of that weren't enough, people who are chronically sleep-deprived actually die younger. That is, those who get an insufficient amount of restorative sleep actually have earlier death rates, from other causes, as compared to those who get a healthy amount of sleep. So not only does a lack of sleep leave you feeling physically and cognitively depleted, but your health—in the most fundamental way—is on the line.

You might have already guessed it, but epigenetics also plays a role in how sleep affects your health. Sleep, just like nutrition and physical activity, has a direct impact on how your genes express themselves. Insufficient sleep leads to negative consequences in your genetics; for instance, poor sleep will lead to you feeling stressed out, thanks to the way certain genes turn on and off. That, in turn, will affect your quality of life and overall health. On the other hand, getting good sleep will lead to better genetic expression: the expression of your best self.

WHAT IS HEALTHY SLEEP?

A healthy person cycles between two different kinds of sleep during the night. There's rapid-eye movement, or REM, sleep, and there's non-REM sleep. Non-REM sleep has three stages. In the first stage, you're not entirely asleep; you're somewhat alert but becoming relaxed. In the second stage you've fallen asleep, your muscles have relaxed, and your brain waves have begun to slow. Then, in stage three, you have what's called slow-wave sleep. This is where your breathing decelerates and your body becomes immobile, and where your body repairs itself and releases growth hormones. All of that is your non-REM sleep. In REM sleep, as its name suggests, your eyes begin to flutter, you dream vividly, and your brain repairs and rebalances itself.

A healthy night's sleep includes both REM and non-REM, because you need both types in order to rebuild yourself. Most people complete a full sleep cycle, with both types of sleep, roughly every 90 to 120 minutes. This varies from person to person, but generally speaking, your body completes a cycle and starts again within that time frame. Over the course of a regular night's sleep, your body goes from cycle to cycle to cycle. Some people need four full cycles in order to repair themselves, while other people need five.

That's why *both* quality and quantity of sleep matter for your health. You might be lying in bed for eight hours, but if you're not getting enough oxygen—like Ryan—and your body is stressing out, then you're not cycling into the deep sleep that actually restores you in body and mind. In the opposite case, people might get really great deep sleep, but if they're only getting four or five hours each night, then their health is still suffering.

SLEEPING DISORDERS AND OUR MODERN WORLD

For most of human history, there was no artificial light. There were fires and torches and candles and gas lamps, yes, but generally speaking, we were more or less awake with the daylight and asleep when it was dark.

And then, suddenly, there were light bulbs. Thanks to that artificial light, we could stay up later.

And in very recent history, the artificial glow of the light bulb was joined by the glow of our televisions, computers, smartphones, and tablets. These new devices emit a certain type of illumination called "blue light" that suppresses our melatonin production. Melatonin is a hormone that's crucial for our circadian rhythms—that is, it's crucial for our natural sleep/wake cycle.

So not only have we left behind the epoch in which sundown was our signal to sleep, but now we sit in bed with our devices. And though we may think that's a good way of relaxing, in fact, what we're doing is making it less likely that we'll be able to fall asleep. That blue light makes us alert. It has that effect even when we're already tired. So there we are, at the moment when we should be going to sleep, and we're unwittingly exposing ourselves to something that will keep us awake.

Our ability to keep our homes illuminated at night, our perpetual busyness, our exposure to information, and our forms of entertainment are all causing the modern trend of disordered sleeping, and that's keeping us from getting the rest we need to be healthy. Our circadian rhythms are very important to our health. We must arrange our waking and sleeping in a manner that supports normal circadian rhythms. I describe this in more detail on our web hub.

DIAGNOSING YOUR SLEEP PROBLEM

If you're suffering from a lack of sleep, you may have what's called "sleep insufficiency syndrome," or you may have insomnia or a related disorder. Here's some brief information on these two different types of conditions.

SLEEP INSUFFICIENCY SYNDROME

The first type of sleep disorder actually does not require visiting a physician. You can manage it in your own home. When individuals suffer from sleep insufficiency syndrome, the problem comes down to the fact that they're not truly giving themselves enough opportunity to sleep.

This may be the case for you, even if you think you really do give yourself sufficient opportunity to sleep. You might be maintaining certain habits that are actually sabotaging your sleep. If that's the case, the recommendations in this chapter will help you to develop new habits that will facilitate good, healthy sleep.

Many people come into my office concerned about their cognitive function and their fatigue, and a quick inventory of their habits reveals they have sleep insufficiency syndrome. I go through a process of confirming that there are no other conditions causing their symptoms, and we settle on the diagnosis: insufficient sleep.

Then they ask me how they can start to feel better—and the first and only answer is *sleep*. Until you give your body and mind the rest that it needs to function, there's nothing else we can do improve your energy or your cognition. Sleep is non-negotiable. If you're not getting enough of it, your productivity will suffer.

INSOMNIA AND RELATED DISORDERS

Unlike sleep insufficiency syndrome, insomnia and related disorders are medical conditions. These imply that you have an inability to get into deep sleep in a timely fashion or that you tend not to cycle through restorative sleep as you're supposed to.

There are many reasons a person might have such a disorder. It could be the result of depression or other mental health issues. It could be a neurochemical issue. It could be the result of working a night shift or a circadian rhythm disorder. It could be due to obstructive sleep apnea, in which you don't breathe well while you're asleep and therefore your body ends up stressed out through the night because it doesn't have enough oxygen. It could be the result of a medication or substance that prevents normal sleep cycling, or a limb movement disorder, or a pain disorder.

If you have a medical condition that is disrupting your sleep, I would strongly recommend that you consider seeing a clinician for a full evaluation in order to diagnose and treat the problem.

TREATING YOUR SLEEP PROBLEM

The appropriate treatment for disordered sleeping depends on the precise nature of the problem. But there are certain things that are applicable to everyone who could use more sleep. Below, you'll find crucial information about the concept of *sleep hygiene* and about developing healthy habits that are conducive to restful, restorative sleep. You'll also find information about cognitive behavioral therapy and about medications for sleep disorders.

SLEEP HYGIENE

As with every health issue that we're tackling in this book, sleeping healthfully has everything to do with habit, awareness, and intentionality. I hope this chapter has already convinced you that getting good sleep is non-negotiable for your health—and because of that, you've already begun to feel a strong desire to focus on your sleep habits, to become aware of those habits, and then to modify those habits to get into a rhythm of restorative sleep. Once you begin to move in that direction, your new habits eventually will become self-perpetuating. Sleeping *well* will become your habit.

The following recommendations for cultivating sleep-friendly habits will be beneficial for *everyone*—whether you're already a good sleeper or you suffer from clinical insomnia. These principles are about getting into good sleep patterns, and in some cases they can be powerful enough for individuals to get over insomnia. That's right: sometimes people can develop such good habits that they overcome their medical diagnosis.

Before we get into the habits themselves, I want to return one more time to the importance of your *thinking*:

- You have to accept that you need sleep. You've got to become *aware* of how a lack of sleep has negative consequences for your health.

- You have to *desire* sleep. Indeed, you have to desire sleep so much that you're willing to change your habits in order to get the sleep you need. Such change must be *necessary*.

- You have to become *aware* of your current habits.

- Finally, you need to develop the *competency* to change your old habits into healthy new ones. The purpose of this chapter is to help you do this.

Once you've gotten your thinking to the right place, it's time to turn to the specific habits that constitute sleep hygiene. *Sleep hygiene* is the idea that you should approach sleep with the kind of intentional routine that you bring to your personal hygiene. You take showers. You brush your teeth. You do these things without thinking about them, and together, they add up to a routine that keeps your body clean. You're now going to learn how to develop a similar routine that facilitates healthy sleep.

The first step in developing sleep hygiene is to understand how your current habits may be keeping you awake. As an example, consider my patient Sally, who came to see me after sleeping well for most of her life. Then she fell into a pattern in which she just couldn't get restful sleep.

"Not only do I have trouble falling asleep," she told me, "but when I do fall asleep, I wake up three hours later and I can't fall back asleep. I've gotten to the point where just getting into bed makes me anxious, because I know I'm going to be lying there worrying about how I can't sleep."

This lack of sleep was affecting Sally in a number of ways. Not only was she exhausted, but the fatigue was beginning to affect her mood. She was worried she was becoming depressed.

To get her started on a solution, we took an inventory of her habits—and I immediately learned how busy Sally is. She works part-time in communications and she's the mother of three. She has a ton of responsibilities. Sally's typical day included checking email and Facebook as soon as she woke up to see what was ahead in the day and what needed her attention. Then she got her kids off to school and went to the office, where she spent her time on the computer and phone. Her office doesn't give her access to natural light while she's there.

Then, in the afternoon, Sally would wrap up work, pick up her kids, and shuttle them to their various activities. She enjoyed this part of her day, she said, which involved socializing with other parents and spending some time outside. Then she went home, fixed dinner with her spouse, helped the kids with homework, and got everyone settled for the night.

As soon as the kids were in bed, Sally would go back to the computer to catch up on whatever she'd missed at the office. Then she and her husband would climb into bed and unwind by watching Netflix. Their favorite show was *Breaking Bad*, which they liked to watch for an hour or two. And just before switching off the light to go to sleep, Sally usually picked up her tablet to check her email one last time.

But when the light finally clicked off, she couldn't sleep.

After assessing her habits to determine how she could develop a routine of sleep hygiene, it was clear that some things about Sally's current routine were out of her control. She couldn't do anything about the fact that she uses a computer at work, nor could she change the lack of natural light in her office. And the fact that she was busy juggling a ton of responsibilities wasn't going to change anytime soon.

But there was still a lot that was within her control. Here are the changes that we devised together.

Sally stopped checking email and Facebook first thing in the morning. She decided she could wait until after she had at least gotten out of bed, gone outside with the family dog, and had a glass of water.

During her workday, she focused on being efficient while she was at her desk, then rewarding herself with short breaks to the part of the building where there are large windows that let in a lot of light. And whenever her schedule would allow it, she started going out for a walk at lunchtime. But even when she doesn't have time for a walk, she now takes at least a few minutes to just sit by the sunny window and *breathe*.

During the afternoon hours, she started intentionally ignoring her smartphone and tablet unless something required her immediate attention. She focused, instead, on simply getting her kids where they needed to go, taking care of her errands, and engaging with the people around her.

In the evenings, she started using her computer only to take care of necessary tasks. She decided she could stop checking her email and Facebook within two hours of getting into bed. On top of that, she and her husband stopped watching *Breaking Bad*, or any other highly stimulating show, on weeknights; they now save that stuff for the weekends. Instead, they watch something mellow, or they read, or they just enjoy catching up with each other.

After she made those changes, it only took Sally a few weeks to start sleeping. And pretty soon, she was getting great sleep. All she had to do was change her habits.

Guidelines for sleep hygiene:

- Avoid stimulants—including caffeine, decongestants, and medications, if possible—after lunchtime. Avoid caffeine within 10 hours of bedtime.

- Exercise. All forms of exercise help to ensure sound sleep. Intensive physical activities should be conducted in the morning or the late afternoon, while relaxing exercises, like yoga, can be done before bed to help initiate restful sleep.

- Soak up some natural light. Exposure to natural light helps maintain normal sleep-wake cycles. Get as much natural light as you can during the day.

- Turn off devices within two hours of bedtime. (I know, I know. Two hours is all the time you have in the evening. But it's your choice. If you want to sleep—and feel healthy—then this is what you've got to do.) Keep your devices at least five feet away from you (preferably more) while sleeping.

- Limit overall exposure to screens. Use blue light blocking programs or glasses. Change out light bulbs in your home to warmer bulbs. As much as possible, minimize your exposure to unnatural light sources.

- Your bed and bedroom should be relaxing and comfortable. You should have a good mattress and pillows.

- Your bedroom should be fully dark; consider it your sleep sanctuary. That might mean purchasing light-blocking curtains, as well as removing any screens or clocks that emit a glow. That light can keep you awake.

- You bedroom must be quiet. If there are surrounding noises coming into your room, you can use a white noise machine or a machine that makes a relaxing sound such as waves on a beach.

- Do *not* sleep with the TV on. In fact, get the TV out of the bedroom altogether.

- Your bed should *not* be the place where you watch movies, watch television, read, work on your laptop, write emails, or check social media. Your bed should be the place where you sleep. This is important because you're teaching your brain to get into a routine. If you use your bed for working or staring at screens, then your brain is going to turn *on* when you get into bed, instead of shutting off.

- You will sleep better if you can keep your bedroom at a cool temperature. Recent studies have revealed that humans sleep more soundly if the environment is cool. Try keeping your bedroom at 67 degrees, if that is possible for you.

It's important to note that *anything* that's emitting an electromagnetic frequency affects our brain and, thus, can affect our sleep. You should not have your cell phone or tablet plugged in beside you. Those devices, even when they're off, give off electromagnetic energy. If you need to use your phone as an alarm clock, it should be five feet away from you. Dim it, and turn it face down.

The wisdom behind these guidelines is a notion of "stimulus control," which simply means that you're going to start taking control of anything that's stimulating you to wake up or stay awake. These guidelines are a program for reversing the habits that are interfering with your sleep in order to train yourself to go to sleep when it's bedtime.

It's generally useful to develop a whole routine that you do each night as you move toward bed. Maybe it's just walking around slowly to turn off lamps and lights. Maybe you switch on a particular music that's relaxing, or you take a hot shower. Some people do a meditation that focuses their breathing. The idea is to help your brain settle down and to do so in a routine that helps your body and mind develop positive habits.

During this evening routine, consider intentionally steering your mind away from thoughts about the day that just ended, or about what's ahead tomorrow, or anything else that might provoke anxiety. Instead, steer yourself toward thoughts and activities that are soothing. This might take some practice. As you catch yourself thinking about work or other responsibilities, just stop and remind yourself that there's nothing you have to do about those things right now. Remind yourself that you'll be prepared for tomorrow when tomorrow comes—and that the best thing you can do right now is rest.

You may also want to use a form of progressive relaxation once you've gotten into bed, in order to continue to steer your thoughts in a soothing direction and away from any worries or anxieties. Once you've closed your eyes, focus on the sensations in your body. Beginning at the top of your head and working your way slowly to your toes, take the time to notice what's happening in each bodily region. Is your jaw clenched? Is there tension in your neck? Notice how it feels to rest on the soft sheets and mattress. (There are many audio resources available that can take you through this type of progressive relaxation in a guided manner.)

As you scan the sensations of your body in this way, breathe deeply, in and out through your nose, and begin to release some of the tension that's present in your muscles. Allow this relaxation to move down your body, from your head into your neck, to your shoulders, into your arms and fingers. See if you can feel the tension leave through your fingertips. Then notice as the relaxation moves through your torso, into your pelvis, down your legs and calves, and see if you can feel tension leaving through your toes.

In this mode of relaxation, you're essentially hypnotizing yourself. You're moving into a relaxed state, which is the pre-stage for sleep.

A slightly different version of this progressive relaxation is to take deep, controlled breaths and to count them, as we described in Chapter Six. And as you do so, count the inhalations and exhalations. Count to ten and then start back at one. Some people also find it helpful to picture themselves in a very relaxed setting—for instance, floating on waves—as they do this, in order to encourage their brain into a very relaxed and pleasurable state.

These techniques are especially helpful for people who suffer from a common ailment that inhibits sleep: a restless mind. Sometimes, it's your thoughts themselves that are preventing you from sleeping. If you're chronically sleep-deprived, your nervousness and worry about not being able to sleep can turn into a major source of anxiety all on its own, which then prevents sleep.

I've had my own troubles with sleep deprivation from a restless mind. (A restless mind, as it turns out, is the most common reason that people end up at the doctor's office with a sleep problem.) When I was training to be a physician, there were times when I had to work 100 hours a week, and that made it hard for me to maintain any kind of healthy sleep routine. Perhaps you've had a similarly difficult period during your professional life.

Then, when I finished my medical training, I started a business at the same time that my wife and I started a family. My perpetual busy-ness, combined with all my anxieties about supporting my new family, began to keep me awake at night.

But that experience is precisely what makes me so confident in the program of sleep hygiene that I'm recommending to you. I follow this same process myself—and it works. Controlled breathing and progressive relaxation techniques are powerful, and they're your route to taming a restless mind. Of course, they may not work the first few times you try them (although they might). It may take some practice, in which you really train your brain. But once you develop a habit of this type of relaxation to facilitate sleep, a worrisome thought or a sudden noise in the middle of the night will no longer be a problem—because now you'll be able to relax yourself and fall back asleep, even in the face of distractions.

COGNITIVE BEHAVIORAL THERAPY/CBT-I

While the habits of sleep hygiene are beneficial for everyone—and will completely solve sleep disorders for most people—some individuals will require additional treatment. Specifically, for those who suffer from a diagnosis of insomnia or a related condition, cognitive behavioral therapy is the treatment most highly recommended by medical professionals. There is good evidence to show its effectiveness, and the evidence even indicates that patients who go through a program of cognitive behavioral therapy often end up being able to solve future sleep problems on their own. What's more, unlike other treatments—such as medication—cognitive behavioral therapy is extremely safe. For anyone seeking medical treatment for a sleep disorder, I would suggest that cognitive behavioral therapy should be the first and primary resource.

In this type of therapy, you develop a habit of thinking, and a habit of approaching sleep, in a way that helps you to become a good sleeper for the rest of your life. It's powerful. And it has little in the way of side effects or potential down sides.

CBT-I seeks to reduce cognitive and physical arousal. It is highly effective. A period of successful sleep initiation and maintenance is important psychologically. It renews confidence in the ability to sleep, which reduces anxiety. CBT-I includes behavioral interventions such as stimulus control and sleep restriction.

With stimulus control, we attempt to eliminate any stimuli that interfere with the mental association between the bed and successful sleep. This is similar to addressing sleep hygiene but goes a little deeper. We suggest that the bed be used only for sleep (and intimacy), and to get out of bed whenever you are awake unless you are clearly about to go to sleep. You should avoid looking at a clock during the night. You should also sleep only in your own bed and in no other places in your home. When combined with a sleep log, this becomes a very effective tool. Many patients find that the behaviors or habits they thought were helping them get some sleep were the very habits that were interfering with their sleep.

Sleep restriction is based on the concept that insomnia causes individuals to spend too much time awake in bed, which creates a conditioned arousal response to the bed. With sleep restriction, we suggest you choose a six-hour window of time that you are allowed to be in bed. We suggest you maintain this schedule for two to four weeks. It's important to note that this approach may actually induce some sleep deprivation in the first few weeks. However, it is a short-term intervention that is designed to change the expectation of nightly insomnia that has been ingrained into your thinking. You definitely should use a sleep log to track your sleep efficiency when using this technique.

Your sleep efficiency is the amount of time you spent asleep versus the total time you spent in bed. For instance, if you spent six hours in bed and slept for four of them, your sleep efficiency would be 4/6, or 67 percent. Once you are achieving a sleep efficiency of 85 percent or greater, you may lengthen your allowed time in bed by 15 minutes each week until you are obtaining seven to nine hours of sleep per night. This can be a very effective technique for breaking the cycle of insomnia.

SLEEP RESTRICTION

1. Choose a six-hour interval. The starting time is the time that you actually get into bed and the end time is when you get up. This may seem like a significant reduction in the time that you allow for sleep, but it will still be more time than you presently spend sleeping.

2. If you find that you are wide-awake during the six-hour interval, get out of bed and conduct a quiet activity. Do not turn on a computer or the television. Consider reading, utilizing a restful meditation, or praying. Only return to bed when you feel drowsy.

3. Maintain a sleep log and track your sleep efficiency. When your sleep efficiency is 85 percent or better, expand your allowed time in bed by 15 minutes each week.

Cognitive behavioral therapy is available via personal interactions with a trained therapist, perhaps near you. It's also available through online portal tools in which you can go through the process without actually going to someone's office.

Some insurance plans cover this type of therapy. If yours does not, it may still be affordable by negotiating a bundle package for the appointments you'll need. But if you seek out this resource and can't find what you need, contact my office. We have a therapist specifically trained in how to help people get care, and we can do virtual visitations for this purpose. So if you feel that you're not going to be able to access this type of resource without help, I would encourage you to contact our organization to see if we can help you. It's that important, and it's really that easy to get started.

In terms of cognitive tools, the breathing and meditation skills from Chapter Six are some of the most powerful techniques out there for becoming a great sleeper. Meditation techniques—which are often recommended by behavioral therapists—help with neuroplasticity and stress control. They can do wonders to help you sleep well every night.

If you find you are not getting sufficient sleep with the techniques we have outlined then please consider maintaining a sleep log. You can find templates for these online at no cost. A sleep log will often reveal obvious behavioral patterns that reinforce insomnia (e.g., spending excessive time in bed, having regular bed/wake times, daytime napping that diminishes sleep ability in the evening). In addition, sleep logs may reveal circadian rhythm disorders that can then be addressed.

SLEEP MEDICATIONS

Many people who have trouble sleeping go into their doctor's office seeking a prescription. Sometimes they've tried Ambien or a similar pill and found that it really helped them, and they often believe that's the best solution.

In fact, though, medication is *not* the medically recommended treatment for sleep disorders—for a number of good reasons. There's substantial evidence to suggest that it's harmful to take sleep medication on a regular basis. What's more, it doesn't improve the problem in the long term. All of the available prescriptions eventually lead you to develop a tolerance to the drug, meaning they become less effective. You then may develop a dependency in which you can't sleep without the drug, and end up having to take a pill every night.

On top of that, most of these drugs have an impact on how you cycle through restorative sleep, and they can end up having a negative impact on the quality of your sleep. Many of them will also leave you with a sort of hangover in the morning that keeps you from feeling good as you start your day. All of these effects are the very opposite of the health you're trying to achieve by reading and following the guidelines of this book.

However, in some cases, people who have become sleep-deprived and are dealing with severe anxiety might find that short-term use of a prescription drug is helpful. If you're in that position, you should contact your physician and discuss the issue. It's possible that a short course of medication in tandem with therapy is the best approach. But your focus should be on developing the habits described in this chapter to become a good sleeper *without* the use of medications.

Some people also use supplements to help them sleep well. These include things like melatonin, magnesium, valerian root, or over-the-counter antihistamines that are sedating. Most of these are not proven to be effective, though certain individuals may say that they work for them. While most of them are relatively safe, there are potential consequences from using them in the long term. A recent report showed that prolonged exposure to medications that have what's called "cholinergic activity"—which include sedating antihistamines—may lead to dementia. There isn't proof of this, but it's worth noting that long-term use of any medication, including over-the-counter meds, may carry unforeseen negative effects.

On the other hand, if you use a sleep aid intermittently and find that it works for you, it's likely that that's okay. To understand what's smartest and safest for your particular situation, I would encourage you to talk with your personal health provider.

STEP INTO THE CONSULTATION ROOM

You've now made some important changes to your habits involving your thinking, your diet, and your physical activity. Those changes have already helped you to feel better.

But you're still struggling with fatigue and some problems with short-term memory, and your mood still isn't as good as you'd like it to be. When you come back to my office for your next appointment, I ask about your sleep habits.

You explain that you try to be in bed by 11, though it's often later. You say that you have trouble falling asleep and you tend to wake up frequently. You have to get up at six. And you report that you almost never feel genuinely rested when you get out of bed.

We discuss the idea of sleep hygiene and you decide to take some initial steps to move yourself toward a healthier sleep regimen. We agree on the following program:

- Though it's hard for you to imagine turning off your devices a full two hours before bedtime, you say that you'll try thirty minutes beforehand, and then see if you can increase it from there.

- You acknowledge that some of the TV shows you watch right before bed might not be the best for helping you relax, and you agree to either watch something calming or nothing at all. You're actually glad to make this change; you say that you weren't really enjoying watching so much TV anyhow. It was just a habit.

- The same goes for caffeine in the afternoon. You used to get a cold Coke to break up your afternoon at work, but you realize that you have no particular attachment to that drink. You decide to switch to seltzer instead.

- You agree to increase your new program of physical activity. On most days, you'll walk briskly for a half hour.

- You agree to get all of the electronics out of your bedroom, except for one device to help you wake up in the morning.

- You also agree to keep practicing the meditation exercises and incorporate breathing techniques to help you relax your brain.

Let's pause here for a moment, because I want to congratulate you. You're tending to a set of issues that are vitally important for your long-term health and that too often go ignored. By doing this work, you'll reap benefits for the rest of your life.

ADDITIONAL RESOURCE

- *Sleep Smarter: 21 Essential Strategies to Sleep Your Way to a Better Body, Better Health, and Bigger Success* by Shawn Stevenson

- SHUTi, an online affordable CBT resource for sleep

- Brain.fm, An app that uses auditory signaling to induce sleep

- Oura Ring, An excellent sleep tracking device

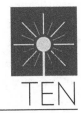

TEN

Purpose: When You Know Why You're Here, You Stick Around Longer

This chapter explores the deepest determinant of health: a sense of your life's purpose. We must feel a sense of purpose in order to engage in all the other habits that support health. Without purpose, we lack the most important motivation for caring for our health in the long term. This chapter offers a starting place to help you identify and nurture your own unique purpose.

EVERYONE HAS A PURPOSE. Every individual ever born had a reason for being born: something good that he or she could bring into this world. But many of us lose sight of that purpose. We might feel too overwhelmed by our daily responsibilities to think about it, or we might have encountered difficult circumstances when we were young that made us focus simply on surviving. Or we might have had our minds cluttered by a culture that's perpetually trying to sell us our identity as a replacement for determining our worth for ourselves.

A recent book called *Tribe*, by Sebastian Junger, explains our sociological desire to feel necessary to something larger than ourselves and connected to the people around us. Junger describes the way that we live in modern society, tucked away in our suburban homes, noting that we have little need for others, and others have little need for us. At the same time, he points out that our culture places value on things like money, status, beauty, and possessions—none of which correlate very well with a deeper sense of well-being or happiness. And from the perspective of our mental health, these are big problems, leading to the widespread depression and even suicide that are so much a part of our modern world.

Junger's book is a modern way of explaining something that many of us feel in our bones: A sense of purpose is vital for a fruitful life. It's also an essential part of becoming a steward of your own health and energy, because without purpose, it's too easy to lose steam in the process of trying to change your behaviors and commit to improving your health.

That's why this chapter asks you to look deeply into some big questions: What are you living for? What are your priorities? What do you want for yourself? You probably didn't intend to become unhealthy; most people don't want to be chronically sick, fatigued, or depressed. But somehow, many of us find our way there, far from what we might say is our purpose. Our goal now is to help you clarify what you truly desire for yourself in a larger sense, so that you move forward guided by what *you* want—not what others are telling you to want or to be.

Many of us pursue temporary identities rather than genuine purpose. Sometimes we do so through our professional lives. We consider our work to be our identity, and that allows us to set aside the larger question of purpose. We actually live in a time when that's very common.

But all of us should take a step back in order to ground ourselves in something more solid. For instance, my work as a physician is only one part of my identity. It's important that I not invest too much of myself in the fact that I'm a doctor, because that professional identity could change. Something could happen that renders me incapable of practicing medicine. And if being a doctor were my entire identity, I would find myself wrecked if such a thing ever happened. I would have an existential crisis wondering who I am. Thus, my identity can't simply be the fact that I'm a physician—or even that I'm a husband and a father. It needs to be founded on what I believe is my eternal essence.

We also have a tendency to seek instant gratification through substances that are supposed to give us an immediate boost in our physical or emotional well-being but actually take us away from our deeper purpose. Many of us take some form of pill or other substance every day because it briefly alters our brain chemistry so that we feel better. But over time, those substances can affect our baseline neurochemistry in such a way that we need the substance simply to maintain a minimum state of comfort. That's led to alarming rates of addiction in our society. We have become enslaved to substances that supposedly promise instant gratification but in fact create an entirely false sense of well-being.

It's also very common in our modern times to create our identities through online social connections. We have a natural need and desire for interaction with others, and social media experiences tap into that and often hold great power over us as a result. The concept of likes and dislikes—and public forums in which we're praised or affirmed or criticized—can be a very dangerous place for the human psyche to live.

You should be aware of how much power these tools have over you, because they can take you away from your present moment and contribute to a sense of insecurity. Such insecurity arises naturally when we don't have a strong sense of who we are, and as we wrestle with it, we find ourselves in a state of perpetual need. We need others to affirm us. We need others to tell us continually that we matter—because we don't have a strong sense of that truth within us.

The companies that are out there trying to sell you their products understand all of that. They employ social and behavioral psychologists and neuroscientists to help them develop marketing strategies based on how people think and what influences us. And when we don't know who we are, in the deepest and truest sense, we're vulnerable to their marketing overtures. We become like conditioned animals, responding to the signals and traps set out for us. We can end up spending a lot of money—sometimes money that we don't even have—to buy things that we think will give us identity, even as they often take away our health, our energy, and the experience of the irreplaceable present.

The truth is that each one of us is in search of our identity, trying to discover and understand who we are and how we fit into the larger world. Most of us are also wrestling with insecurities related to that. We're not sure if we matter. We're not sure if we have value. In some ways, this is yet another feature that distinguishes our modern world from past eras, in which people's roles within their families often gave them a clear purpose. In the present day, we tend to be much more financially comfortable, so we don't always need to focus on our family's immediate survival. For most people in this country today, our basic needs are met. Our deepest needs, however, go neglected.

Our deepest needs are to know that we matter and to know that there's something about life that's worth showing up for. When *those* needs are met, we see that each day is an opportunity to experience life fully and to take another step forward in our unique service to the world. But the only way to gain access to that deeper sense of meaning is to move beyond the constant pursuit of temporary identity by having a strong internal sense of who you are and what your life is about.

Indeed, true contentment comes not through a professional identity, and certainly not through substances or social media, but in connecting with people we love and in talking with them about the things that matter. It comes through developing a sense of responsibility around who we are and what we're doing, and then pursuing it.

For many people, genuine contentment also comes through a fundamental belief system, whether it's religious or spiritual or philosophical. Most people have some belief system, whether they're aware of it or not. And so, as you move into this work of considering and identifying your life's purpose, it's important to take the time to reflect on what you believe. What concepts and values do you feel are eternal and thus transcend your individual life? What do you believe about life and death and whatever may come after? A belief system, whatever it is, can serve as an anchor and will allow you to approach the question of purpose from a position of strength and courage.

It's also true that there are no formulas through which you can identify your purpose. No one can tell you what your purpose is; that's for you to determine. The strategies and modes of thinking that I've collected into this chapter are intended to inspire you in the right direction, but only you can pick up the threads and weave them into a sense of unique purpose for your own life. In fact, one of your great quests in this life is to figure out your purpose and then to live in accordance with it.

As you begin to consider these profound questions and to gain clarity around who you are and what your life is about, it will then become easier for you to align your daily habits with your larger goals. You'll have a growing sense of what you genuinely desire, and that will make it more likely that you'll start to maintain good habits that support you in body and mind—first as you walk the road back to good health, and then onward through the rest of your life, as you manifest your unique purpose.

STRATEGIES AND TOOLS FOR IDENTIFYING AND CLARIFYING YOUR PURPOSE

◆ Start by taking some notes

This process of searching out your purpose requires posing questions that may be unfamiliar terrain for you. Why am I here? What do I believe in? What's most important to me? What are my greatest priorities? Consider each of these questions in turn, and allow yourself to pause, especially as you come across questions and concepts that are new to you and provoke thought. Breathe deeply. Let your brain dwell in these questions and, perhaps, in the ambiguity that arises. Then start to take notes about this process and the responses that come to mind.

Throughout this book, we've emphasized awareness—of your thinking, your emotions, and your actions. One of the most effective tools in the pursuit of awareness is journaling.

There's no specific correct way to keep a journal; it can be electronic, or old-fashioned with a pencil and paper. It can even be a spreadsheet where you make a note of key points about your thinking, your emotions, your actions, and your nutrition. No matter which format is most comfortable for you, the act of journaling is key. Dive deeply into yourself and write down what you find.

WRITE ABOUT YOUR PAST—AND THEN YOUR FUTURE

Begin to reflect on your past by going decade by decade through your life. This might seem painstaking and challenging, but it's well worth the effort. For each decade, write down what you remember. Not every memory, but the big memories. Try also to recall and record any associated sensory experience—how things smelled, tasted, and looked, like the sun in the sky or the color of a parent's jacket. Those sensory memories are very powerful.

There are a few reasons to do this exercise. First of all, you're collecting your memories so that you'll have them in the future, because we forget more and more as time passes. But you're also recording these key moments of your life in order to understand how they affected you. How did these various experiences lead you to form attachments and your sense of yourself? Some will be positive, others negative. Go decade by decade. At the end of each decade, look at it as a whole and try summing it up. Think about how it influenced who you are, for better or worse. Then move on to the next decade, all the way to where you are now. You'll find that you understand yourself and why you do the things you do more clearly.

As you go through this exercise, you're likely to encounter experiences that were painful, either in a physical or an emotional sense. Most of us have experienced things that were out of our control and that left us injured in deep ways. It can be painful to think deeply about your story and to revisit things that you may regret or that shaped you in ways you lament.

But as we talked about back in Chapter Four, the present moment shouldn't be held hostage to the past, regardless of what occurred. Your task now is to acknowledge the past in order to understand how it made you who you are, and then to live fully here in the present by taking control of your habits and shaping them in ways that nourish and energize you. Right now, your future is undecided, and you're the one who will decide it. Claiming ownership over your future also includes reconciling the past.

It may be the case that there are such traumatic experiences in your past that you're not able to surmount them on your own. That's the case for many of us. If it's true for you, then I would strongly encourage you to work with a professional counselor who's trained in helping people who have post-traumatic stress disorder (PTSD) or a related condition. Working with such a counselor is *not* a sign of weakness—on the contrary, it's like hiring a personal trainer. Your counselor is someone who will help you approach life from the strongest possible standing.

Once you've done the exercise of recalling and recording key moments from the past, turn your sights on the future. Begin to consider what you want your legacy to be. Imagine writing your autobiography. Make notes about what you want it to say. Or write your eulogy. What do you want people to say about you when you're no longer around? How do you want to be remembered? What kind of legacy do you hope to leave behind? This is often a fruitful way of examining what matters most to you, because it tends to clear away the clutter of our daily lives and lets us examine only what's most important. These are your ultimate priorities.

Let those priorities illuminate the way toward the habits and actions that will help you achieve your goals. Ask yourself, how are you going to get from where you are now to where you want to be in the end? Write it down.

INTEGRATE YOUR LEFT AND RIGHT BRAIN

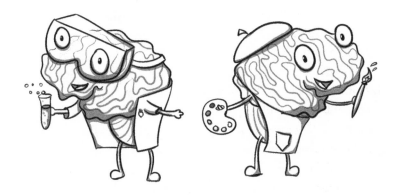

Each of us has a left-brain and a right-brain hemisphere. In order to simplify a pretty complicated topic, we'll simply say that the left brain is your deductive, scientific, and linear brain. It's how you put together two and two to get four. It does your concrete thinking. Your right brain is your creative and artistic side; it's the part of your brain that's capable of envisioning and imagining things that don't exist or aren't right in front of you. Both sides of your brain are involved in regulating your emotions, but often, the right side is referred to as the emotional regulator. It is important to understand that the brain is more integrated than I describe here.

Thanks to our genetic predisposition as well as our life experiences, we usually develop a tendency to be either far more left-brained or far more right-brained. Left-brained people tend to be very straightforward and pragmatic. They seem less emotional. They try to identify solutions in a given moment, and they become uncomfortable in situations that are not concrete for them. They generally do not excel at communication, especially emotional communication, and they tend not to be as good at understanding how important emotions are to the human experience.

In fact, left-brainers are often a bit afraid of emotions. This can cause them to try to escape when they encounter emotional or creative thinking, which in turn can create conflict in their relationships and in their lives. By contrast, people who are very right-brained can come across as irrational and unfocused.

Nearly all of us would benefit from better integration of these two hemispheres of the brain. By working toward such integration, you'll develop a powerful toolkit for pursuing your life's purpose as well as your health: the ability to think in a concrete, linear fashion, plus the ability to be creative and imaginative, with a sense of intimate connection to your feelings and emotions.

Thanks to neuroplasticity, such integration is within reach for all of us. Recall from Chapter Four that there are three types of activities that enhance neuroplasticity and help us grow new neural networks: (1) sustained aerobic activity; (2) exercises to improve focus; and (3) novel learning experiences. I'm emphasizing this again because *all three types of activity* are absolutely essential for your ability to stimulate new neural activity and growth and for pruning neural networks that are not useful to you.

If you feel that you're mostly a left-brain person and you'd like to be more creative, consider reading poetry, listening to new types of music, and attending art shows. For decades, even centuries, our culture has emphasized logic and the left brain over creativity and the right brain; we have perhaps focused too much on ordering and classifying and putting everything into scientific boxes.

Personally, I'm much more of a left-brain thinker, which makes me a capable physician. But I've found, as I've matured, that I place great value on exposing myself to music and poetry and art, and on stopping to appreciate how much creative and emotional expression there is in those art forms. Taking the time to interpret those expressions of another person's mind actually helps the two sides of my brain to integrate. I become a better thinker—and a more creative thinker—by exposing myself to creativity.

On the other hand, if you tend to be creative but have a harder time with logical thinking, it's important for you to develop your working memory and executive functions, to focus on categorizing things and putting them together in a logical way. While our culture has in the past placed perhaps excessive emphasis on scientific logic, the very recent phenomenon of mobile devices and social media is rapidly reducing our ability to do focused work.

Multitasking while engaging with social media platforms can negatively impact executive functions of the brain. This phenomenon has been accompanied by a rise in symptoms associated with attention deficit disorder (ADD), including in adults. Adults who were never diagnosed with this problem in early life are now finding that they can't focus their brains. It's essential that we spend time developing our brain's executive function and organization; without these skills, it's difficult to interpret the circumstances around us correctly and to make rational choices in response. There are resources to help you with this at the end of the chapter.

MEDITATE TO ACCESS YOUR WITNESS

One of the most powerful tools for tapping in to your deeper purpose is the type of meditation that we discussed in Chapter Six.

Sit quietly. Breathe deeply and turn your attention to your breath. Spend some time counting your breaths until you've cleared away the monkey brain. And then allow your witness, your intuitive brain, to turn on. Picture yourself in a restful, restorative place, whether it's on a beach, or at a lake, or in a meadow, or in any place that's personally significant to you. Take the time to appreciate the beauty of that place. Imagine yourself feeling completely at peace exactly where you are.

Now, from that feeling of peacefulness, extend a sense of compassion toward others. Focus on a feeling of compassion for someone you love, perhaps in particular for someone who's facing a difficult challenge in his or her life.

Next try to do the same thing for someone you don't know very well—perhaps someone who sold you coffee this morning, or bagged your groceries. Send that person all the compassion and peace that you've summoned in this meditative state.

Next, if you're feeling up to it, try doing the same thing for someone who you find difficult. Set aside those hard feelings and focus simply on sending that person compassion and forgiveness.

Finally, take the time to extend that feeling inward. See if you can summon a great sense of compassion for yourself, exactly as you are. Give yourself a gentle reminder that you matter, and your life has purpose.

When you emerge from this meditative state, notice whether you feel restored or in any way different from how you felt before.

This type of meditation can be a powerful way to begin truly to know yourself. It's a way to recognize some of the different voices that accumulate in your head: the voices that make you feel shame, guilt, remorse, anger, or jealousy. We all have those voices that tend toward a negative interpretation of our life experiences. Going into this meditative place allows us to reshape that interpretation in a positive way.

Such meditation also has real and positive effects on your brain function—effects that scientists have captured through neuroimaging. When scientists look at the brain of someone who has entered into a meditative state, they see that the prefrontal cortex begins to light up with activity; they can actually *see* the higher brain turn on.

They can also see the neurological effects when a person is stuck in negative thinking. When individuals live in a state of self-pity, jealousy, or victimhood, their brains actually contract. They operate with far less capacity, using fewer neural networks in their thinking. Their neurons and the communication fibers that extend from them actually look like they're tangled up in thorns. They're wrapped around themselves.

But when such individuals emerge from the negative thinking loop and move into a positive place, it's possible to see how their neurons communicate differently. They form a new neural network that looks like a blossoming tree.

Give yourself that gift by taking the time and space to enter into a meditative state on a regular basis and to move yourself toward the positive.

REFLECT ON THE POSITIVE AND NEGATIVE ASPECTS OF YOUR MIND STATE

As I noted above, the practice of meditating allows you to key into the negative voices that accumulate in your head. Those voices tend to facilitate harmful mindsets such as fear and shame. The psychiatrist David Hawkins created what are called the stages of consciousness, a list of both positive and negative emotions, and proposed that we should focus on dwelling in a state of positive thinking and moving continually upward toward greater positive energy. Here are his categorizations of the stages of consciousness.

Positivity (from moderate to greatest energy):

1. Courage

2. Trust

3. Optimism

4. Forgiveness

5. Acceptance

6. Reverence/ love

7. Joy/ serenity

8. Peace/ bliss

Negativity (from low to lowest energy):
1. Pride/ scorn

2. Anger/ hate

3. Desire/ craving

4. Anxiety

5. Grief/ regret

6. Apathy/ despair

7. Guilt/ blame

8. Shame/ humiliation

Think about the direction in which your own mindset tends to lean. Do you tend to feel optimistic? Perhaps you tend to feel guilty or angry, driven by cravings. Consider what might be at the root of that mindset. Are you hanging on to experiences or influences that would be better discarded? If so, this may be another area in which a professional counselor could be useful to you.

Try, too, to key into any areas where you're maintaining what I call a limiting belief. Limiting beliefs are thoughts like "I can't focus"; "I can't read poetry"; "I'm not good at science"; or, more generally, "I'm not good at [fill in the blank]." All of these statements are fundamentally untrue. Everyone has the ability to increase their competency in new areas—whether those areas are creative or logical—to the extent that they truly desire it.

To succeed, we must discard our limiting beliefs. As you come across your limiting beliefs in the course of your regular daily activities, and as you attempt to develop yourself in new areas, try overriding those negative emotions with a positive statement about your capabilities ("I *can* focus";

"I *am* good at [fill in the blank].")

Your goal is to move out of the negative and into the positive, and toward greater and greater positive energy. Ultimately, you want to feel that you're receiving a strong, internal affirmation that you're loved and cared for and that you matter. Then bring that affirmation into your life as you move through each day, and let it help you as you seek to make positive, healthy choices.

USE THE STRENGTHSFINDER AND OTHER TOOLS

There are numerous additional tools that can help you through this process. As one example, the Gallup Strengths Center has something called the StrengthsFinder tool. It's a simple, evidence-based assessment that you can purchase for a minimal cost. It will identify your five strongest personality categories from a huge spectrum of possibilities. Understanding your strengths ultimately will allow you to arrange your life around them so that you don't feel stuck in your weaknesses, but rather focused on building and amplifying your strengths. Another tool to consider is the Enneagram, a model of the human personality that helps us to understand ourselves through nine different-yet-interrelated personality types.

There are many other good, objective tools besides the StrengthsFinder. You'll find a list of them at the end of the chapter. Use them as a way of getting to know yourself better and thus moving forward on your journey toward individual purpose.

KNOW OTHERS—AND ALLOW YOURSELF TO BE KNOWN

This exploration of purpose isn't meant to be something that you do alone. As you engage in this process, it's critical for you to feel that you know others fully and allow yourself to be known in the same way. You should have people in your life with whom you can communicate honestly; you need to feel that you're listened to and understood, and that you're listening to others and understanding them in kind.

Practice becoming a compassionate listener, and learn to receive compassionate listening from those around you. This might feel uncomfortable at first, because it means sitting in the presence of another human being and truly listening rather than forming our own responses. Being able to focus yourself solely on listening—and listening compassionately—is an important skill. It's also the way to cultivate relationships in which others listen compassionately to you in return.

Consider the doctor/patient relationship as one example. Modern medicine now underemphasizes listening to—and, thus, sensing and feeling—the patient. Our medical system prioritizes data collection and coding. This means that often, the doctor in an exam room is looking at her computer instead of at the patient. But how can that doctor genuinely feel a patient she's not even looking at?

Many people end up feeling dissatisfied with their physicians. It's true that doctors have very little time to engage with each patient, but studies have shown that it actually doesn't take long for patients to get the type of interaction they desire; instead, what matters is that they believe they were listened to and *felt*.

Simply put, our minds are meant to engage with other minds. We're built to engage with one another in an authentic manner, using both left and right brain, to both know and feel. So the next time you're in a conversation—perhaps in a few minutes from now, when you close this book and go on to your next activity—consider keeping your phone tucked inside a pocket. Focus on giving the other person your whole and undivided attention.

If you have a spouse or partner, consider that one of the best roles of a life partner is to embark together on this profound journey of purpose. Genuine partners help one another to better understand themselves, and then hold each other accountable for continuing to grow and become better. True intimacy lies in transparently knowing each other and being co-committed to each other's purpose. When you have a long-term intimate relationship of this nature, it provides you with a source of great stability as you pass through the uncertainties of life.

IT'S THE JOURNEY THAT MATTERS

There is no endpoint or arrival in this process of searching out your purpose—it's a journey that lasts your entire life, and it's the journey itself that matters. Each moment in which you choose something better for yourself matters. Each day you spend tending toward your inner purpose—because you believe you're part of something greater—matters.

There are no shortcuts on this road, and there shouldn't be. Shortcuts imply that the journey is something to be avoided. A popular term these days is "hack"—you can hack your sleep or hack your professional life. I understand why it's an attractive term, but please don't think of your purpose and your health from the standpoint of hacks. You need *real* sleep. You need *real* nutrition. You don't want to hack your way to a less flabby body; you want to possess a genuinely healthy body. Hacks imply taking a shortcut to avoid the journey—when the journey is where all the good stuff happens.

But by now, all of that may be obvious to you. At this point, you may be very clear that you don't want a shortcut or a hack of any kind, because you're keying into your deeper purpose in this life, and you're starting to feel passionate about that purpose.

As that happens, you'll naturally find yourself doing everything in your power to move toward your purpose rather than away from it. You won't be willing to give away your purpose for cheap products. You're going to eat nutritious foods so that you'll have the energy you need to tackle each day. You're going to make sure to get good sleep to restore your brain and elevate your thinking. And you're going to feel less stressed as you start to view the challenges in your path as opportunities to grow and become stronger. You'll find yourself listening to your own body and your own mind and your own heart.

STEP INTO THE CONSULTATION ROOM

You've recently made some major changes with respect to your eating habits, exercise, sleep, and now stress management, and though you've really focused on maintaining a positive outlook—which has helped you to feel more energy as you go about your day—you haven't completely resolved this problem of what seems to be a low-level depression. You come back in to my office for a check-up appointment.

You report that you're sleeping better at night and feeling a lot less pain in your body. You now play outside with your kids on a regular basis, which you really enjoy. You've begun doing the controlled breathing exercises each morning and evening, and you find that they help to calm your worrying mind.

But you're still struggling with motivation for tasks at work and at home, and you wonder if there's still a medical condition that needs to be addressed.

We start to talk about the idea of a deeper purpose. Immediately, the idea resonates with you. You've found the recent changes to your habits and lifestyle to be profoundly beneficial, and this feels like a natural last step in regaining your health. You start to think about how you might make some changes to orient yourself toward what's truly meaningful to you.

Together, we decide that you'll start this process by taking the following action steps:

- Make some notes about your belief system, whether it's religious, spiritual, philosophical, or something else.

- Jot down some notes about what you want in your autobiography or eulogy.

- Journal about some of your personal goals and desires. If you feel comfortable doing so, discuss them with your partner or a friend.

- Consider working with a counselor or coach who shares your faith orientation. Or if you feel that you've experienced profound trauma from events that happened earlier in your life, seek out a therapist who will help you work through these deep-seated issues.

- Try the StrengthsFinder tool and the Enneagram.

- Take five minutes to retreat into a quiet space for some meditative reflection.

- Take another five minutes to think openly and creatively about your purpose. Visualize the destiny you want for yourself.

- If you find parts of this process uncomfortable, experiment with simply sitting with that discomfort, rather than trying to avoid it.

- Make one concrete step in the direction of something you value deeply, whether it's getting involved with a local charity, spending more time with your loved ones, starting a new creative endeavor, or something else.

ADDITIONAL RESOURCES

- *Relevance* by Lee Thayer
- *The Road Back to You: An Enneagram Journey to Self-Discovery* by Ian Morgan Cron and Suzanne Stabile
- *Man's Search for Meaning* by Viktor Frankl
- *The 7 Habits of Highly Effective People* by Stephen Covey

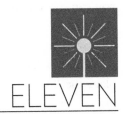

ELEVEN

The Payoff

EVERY CHAPTER OF this book has been grounded in a single notion: your thinking determines your being. Your thinking determines your habits, which determines what you do—and that determines what you're experiencing. That's why, before we got into nutrition guidelines or an exercise regimen, we focused on understanding your brain and becoming intentional about your thinking—so that you'll have the clarity as well as the ability to move toward health.

From there, we did get into authentic nutrition and the importance of movement. We made the important connection between the foods you eat and the energy you feel in your body each day—because the latter arises directly from the former. We covered how to source your foods correctly, how to deal with your appetite, and how to take back control of your choices.

Then we got into a routine for physical movement and biomechanical health. We chucked the concept of fad programs and six-pack abs in favor of knowing the simple truth about your body—that you have to move, and that you have to protect your biomechanics by holding your body in an intentional way.

We talked about how to get the restorative sleep you need in order to open up your brain, clear away old baggage, and feel emotionally and cognitively healthy as you start each day.

We also covered the importance of taking control of your emotional states by using breathing and meditation techniques. I hope you've begun to incorporate those techniques into your life—perhaps even on a daily basis—in order to make intentional stress mastery a core habit. Eventually, you'll get to a place where, whenever you feel stressed, you automatically take a few deep breaths and clear away the monkey brain. From there, you can make conscious choices for yourself, rather than choices based in anger or fear. If already you've begun this habit, then you've likely come a long way from where you started.

There will always be arguments about which is the "best" nutrition plan, the "best" form of meditation, and the "best" way to get a good night's sleep. Those debates will continue. But ultimately, by knowing yourself and your body, you'll know the truth. It's self-evident that eating natural, healthy foods in the right portions; intentionally managing your emotional states; getting good, restorative sleep; moving your body; and focusing on your core purpose are all ingredients for genuine health.

There's just no debating those foundational principles. Look at each of these habits as no different from breathing air, because you can't get by without them.

THE PAYOFF

So what's the ultimate payoff for all this hard work? The payoff is *you*: a healthy, energized, fully alive *you*. And that, of course, means that the payoff is individualized. It will look different for each of us, because each of us wants something different for ourselves. Only you can know how much potential is inside you and what future you desire for yourself.

You stand now at a crossroads. If you're truly sick, or truly hurting, and you continue to maintain the same habits you've always had, then you can expect to continue to be sick and in pain. Our larger healthcare system and an encyclopedia of medications can't do more than palliate your symptoms.

Ultimately, it's up to you.

The payoff is for those who truly desire to be well. If that's you, then the truths presented in this book are a straightforward pathway toward health and vitality.

TURN YOUR FOCUS TO THE FUTURE YOU WANT FOR YOURSELF

Don't let this day end without doing the following exercise.

Get into a comfortable position, calm your breathing, and begin to count your breaths. Clear away your monkey brain and allow your witness to turn on. Then begin to visualize the future you want. This future is your payoff. Exactly what does it look like? How alive and engaged are you with the world around you? Who are you to your family, and within the causes and organizations you care about? What purposes have you dedicated yourself to?

Once you've summoned this picture, let yourself dwell there. Allow yourself to feel it and absorb it, and begin to believe it. Recall the message of epigenetics that we've touched on throughout this book: Our DNA expresses itself based on what we think, what we eat, and how we move through our environment. We are literally creating our destiny through the habits that we cultivate.

For millennia, the gurus of spirituality and philosophy have given us a consistent message: if you strongly desire a particular future, and you enter into deep, contemplative states in which you positively envision that future, you will usually find yourself arriving there. We become what we think about. It may not look exactly as we pictured when we arrive, of course—and unexpected things happen—but overall, we tend to realize what we envision. This is your chance.

START NOW—AND CONTINUE, NO MATTER WHAT

Start now—*right* now. Each step forward matters, no matter how small. Take a step now—whether it's literally taking a step and going outside for a walk, or it's committing to getting a good night's sleep by turning off your devices, or it's choosing not to snack. The key is to start today, and to remember that each step matters.

One of the problems with popular exercise and diet fads is that they tend to promise results in a short time frame—90 days, say. An infomercial promises six-pack abs in 90 days and shows the "before" and "after" pictures to prove it. And in a burst of motivation, we buy whatever product they're selling because we want those abs, too.

But then we have just 90 days to get there. And the program turns out to be more challenging than anticipated—after all, it's difficult to change habits so quickly—and we start to fall behind. We don't see any immediate results, and pretty soon, we quit altogether.

There are a few reasons that this type of program usually fails. The first reason is that we're attempting to put a whole lot of effort into something that's essentially a shallow desire: six-pack abs. For most of us, that's not a serious enough goal to keep us motivated, especially when other influencers—like habit—are so powerful.

But the other problem is the narrow timeframe. Most people need to take baby steps over a long period of time to really change their behaviors and see physical results. Often, the time limit is what dooms these programs to failure. If the advertisements said something like, "Work up to this, and do it for 365 days, and see if you don't look and feel better," people would have a much better chance at succeeding. But of course, that's not a catchy marketing line.

The program in this book isn't meant to be implemented in just 90 days, or 120 days, or even over six months; it's meant to be implemented for your whole life. You haven't failed if you miss a day of exercise or a day of meditation. Instead, you gradually become aware of your habits and, at each turn, you try to do a little bit better.

Perhaps this week you manage one minute of meditation a day. That's all you can do. Next week, it's two minutes. The following week, it's ten. And three years from now, you find yourself meditating for up to an hour—but spread out at different times throughout the day. Perhaps you also find yourself using meditation to improve your sleep, to relax in stressful moments, and to heighten your sense of focus for your purpose.

And maybe you do the same thing with exercise. Maybe you walked for ten minutes today, but in a couple weeks, you start to get into the habit of walking for twenty minutes—and you find yourself really enjoying it. Maybe you end up running a 5K, like my patient Melissa, whom we'll talk about below.

Then you start to make a habit of spending a few minutes on exercises for core strength. And in a few years, it's hard for you to remember that there was a time before you did these things. Start today—and decide you will continue, regardless of setbacks. Start today.

HOW IT'S WORKED FOR A FEW INDIVIDUALS
WHO HAVE COME BEFORE YOU

It might be useful for you to hear the stories of some real people who've been down this road, and how it changed their lives. So the final pages of this chapter are devoted to the stories of Beth, Joe, Melissa, and Steven.

When Beth first came into my office, she described her ailments as pain in her muscles, joints, and back, and well as daily headaches and frequent migraines. She also slept poorly, suffered from low-level depression, and felt chronic fatigue. She was on a constellation of medications to reduce pain and improve sleep because she had previously been diagnosed with fibromyalgia, migraines, tension headaches, insomnia, and moderate persistent depression. The medications helped her some, but not a lot.

Beth works in an office at a computer and is mostly sedentary. She enjoys her work. She also has a supportive family with whom she enjoys spending time, though there are various stressors associated with her family that occasionally trouble her.

When I first met with Beth, we reviewed her medications and concluded that although the prescriptions had helped her at first, they seemed no longer to be working. We reviewed some of the new options on the market, but for various reasons, including undesirable side effects, we decided the newer pharmaceutical options were not a good fit for her.

We started talking about her habits. Her diet consisted of a lot of processed foods, poorly produced meats, and mass-produced vegetables. She had tried a few times to reduce her consumption of sugar and gluten, but that hadn't left her feeling any better. She said she didn't exercise because she felt too tired and her body hurt too much. She didn't have any particular stress-management techniques except to try to spend time with friends and family.

Beth's routine was to wake in the morning, eat cereal, go to work, snack throughout the day, do her computer tasks to the best of her ability, come home, be with her family, watch television, and then try to sleep, though she usually slept fitfully and woke up often.

We began to talk about the importance of restorative sleep to ease her migraines and fibromyalgia and how studies have shown that restorative sleep is one of the most effective interventions. We talked through a basic regimen for improving her sleep.

We also discussed the specific foods she was consuming and identified that many of them could be contributing to inflammation, fatigue, and the fact that she was overweight. We talked about how even ten minutes of very simple physical activity and becoming biomechanically aware could engage her muscles in such a way that she might have less pain and greater strength. We talked about how muscles that are inactive can actually signal to the brain that they're sore or weak, and how that might be part of her discomfort.

So Beth started on some basic interventions. She began a daily ten-minute program of stretching and breathing. She started sourcing her foods a little better. And she started to work on some controlled breathing techniques to help her relax and sleep.

One year later, Beth reported that she was sleeping well. She now rarely had migraine headaches, though she still had tension headaches. She had improved her posture at work. She was having less neck and back pain. She was definitely more flexible and mobile, and she was capable of exercising thirty minutes a day; she said the exercise definitely helped her to feel better. Her energy levels had improved, though she frequently felt tired. And while she was still lacking motivation and energy, she said she felt a bit more hopeful.

At this point, we were able to reduce some of her medications. We also further improved her nutrition plan and got her into a healthier rhythm of eating at meal times with less snacking. We advanced her physical activity routine, and I encouraged her to practice more controlled breathing. We also talked about focusing on a sense of purpose.

Now, two years after that initial visit, Beth reports a much lower level of muscle pain. She has infrequent headaches. She sleeps well most nights. Her energy is good. She has reengaged in many community activities that she enjoys. She's still a little overweight and still deals with intermittent flare-ups of fibromyalgia, but she combats her discomfort with healthier routines. She's on minimal medications.

A couple of years ago, Beth thought that there weren't any solutions out there for her—but her life looks entirely different today. She's satisfied. Her family has observed a major difference in her mood and her positivity. Beth describes her quality of life as very good.

Joe was a really different case. Joe was a middle-aged mechanic with about forty pounds of extra weight around his belly when he first visited my office. He was drinking six beers every night to relax, but he'd never had any problems arise from his drinking; he tried to be very responsible and had no criminal issues. He also used tobacco.

Joe said he didn't eat breakfast or much in the way of lunch. At dinner, though, he ate a whole lot of food, and generally not very good food. He was open about that.

Joe said he had chronic low-back pain and felt tired a lot of the time, although he's tough and not one to complain about his ailments. He said he felt angry about the state of the economy and the elections and various laws that he felt invaded his privacy.

He had high blood pressure that was not well controlled, high tri-glycerides, pre-diabetes, and chronic reflux, for which he had to take pow-erful acid suppressors regularly. He was also on a pain medication that didn't help him a whole lot. Overall, Joe didn't feel good at all.

One of his previous doctors had prescribed him hydrocodone for pain. When he'd switched doctors, the new doctor refused to continue the prescription. Joe doesn't trust doctors.

"I don't want more hydrocodone anyway," Joe had said when the doc-tor refused him the prescription, "because it wasn't working. I just want my pain to go away." Joe can't even take basic ibuprofen, because it gives him stomach ulcers.

When Joe came into my office, one of the first things we looked at was the role of his diet in his physical discomfort, and the fact that his reflux medication—which allowed him to continue eating unhealthy foods—was potentially causing painful side effects. We also talked about how the six beers each night were keeping him from getting restorative sleep. I told him that, if he could cut back even to three beers each night, he would probably sleep a bit better and lose some weight.

What Joe really wanted was to ease his back pain. We explained that the forty pounds around his belly—which he was carrying around all day in his physical job as a mechanic—were the primary cause of his back pain. After taking X-rays, we concluded that there was nothing about his condition that wasn't reversible, because he was mainly suffering from muscle strain.

After his initial appointments, Joe started to believe that his diet and drinking, as well as his lack of sleep and body habits, might be the source of his problem. He started to believe he actually could feel better, and he started to want that for himself.

Still, he was slow and deliberate in making changes to his life and habits. In the first year, Joe slowly reduced his beer consumption from six to three a night, though he often drank more on the weekends. He started trying the exercises we gave him to stretch out his hamstrings and hips and to strengthen his core.

He also started to improve his eating habits. Instead of eating only dinner, he began eating two meals a day, and he changed some of his choices to source his foods a bit better. Joe even brought his wife into our office—because she's the one who does the grocery shopping—so we could tell her how to shop for him. Since Joe is a meat-and-potatoes guy, we showed him how to eat in that way while still getting the right kinds of nutrients.

Joe started to sleep a little better. His mood improved. He started exercising more.

One year after he began making these changes, he was still on blood pressure medication and a prescription for his reflux, and he was still using muscle relaxers for his back pain. He was still frustrated and angry about the state of the world.

Two years out, Joe rarely drinks beer anymore. He's realized that it actually doesn't make him feel any better and that it was just a habit. He's lost twenty of the forty pounds he needs to lose. His back pain is a lot better. Every morning, he does a fifteen-minute workout with his wife that's designed to stretch their bodies and improve their core strength so they can both be healthier.

Joe is now eating in a much healthier way, and he says that his energy has improved. He's cut his reflux medication in half. He's no longer pre-diabetic and he has normal triglycerides. We still treat his blood pressure, though, and he hasn't quit tobacco yet, though he hopes to one day.

Next year, we're hoping that Joe can lose ten more pounds, quit tobacco, and come off his reflux medication altogether. But in the meantime, he reports that he feels a whole lot better. In many ways, Joe is a different person from who he'd been when I first met him.

Then there's the story of my patient Melissa. Melissa is the office manager at a busy doctor's office. She is short in stature and has been severely obese for years. Her work is sedentary and very stressful, and she's gone through a number of significant family stressors over the past several years that adversely influenced her health. Melissa has multiple sclerosis and has been treated for it with various medications.

When I first started working with Melissa, she was frequently sick, often coming in for sinus infections and other maladies. She was generally tired, her body hurt, and she could not lose weight. Though she had always been heavy, she said she was athletic as a child, and her current physical health was nothing like it should have been, based on her own history.

Despite her chronic disease and other challenges, she continued to work hard and to engage in life in a meaningful way. She had purpose, but she lacked the physical health to engage with her purpose in the way she wanted to. She was committed to working on her health until she got better.

The last thing you would have predicted for Melissa was that she would take up running as a way of addressing her issues. She was significantly overweight, with poor posture from her sedentary work, and on medications for a serious chronic autoimmune disorder—hardly an obvious candidate for running. But she decided to enroll in a "couch to 5K" program. She followed the step-by-step process: first walking, then jogging, until at last she completed her 5K. At that point, she felt so good that she began to use Weight Watchers to track her nutrition. She also drew on some of the resources my office gave her to help her choose foods wisely.

When I saw Melissa recently, I learned that she's now in a running club and she's planning for races of longer distances. She's no longer on her medication for reflux, and we had to stop her blood pressure medication because her blood pressure has decreased so markedly. We haven't seen her for an infection in months. Her pain is far less than it was, her energy has improved, she's sleeping better, and her mental clarity is great. She feels alive. She also feels determined to continue to improve her health, and even potentially to reduce the impact that MS has on her body and her daily life.

Melissa has lost fifty pounds. Her BMI still suggests that she's still significantly obese—but we're not really worried about that. We're focused on the fact that she feels good, she's healthier, she has good conditioning, and she's eating healthy foods. She just needs to keep doing what she's doing.

Steven's case is very different from those of Beth, Joe, and Melissa. Steven had opened a Pilates studio in my town and was a health nut. He was fanatical about what he ate and how he exercised and how his body felt and looked. He had lots of tattoos and piercings. He was a very passionate man.

Steven had a couple of chronic conditions that were beyond his control, including asthma that would flare up from time to time and for which he required treatment. Other than that, he was in pretty good health—but he would occasionally experience symptoms including headaches, palpitations, and nervousness, and he would become afraid that he was about to have a dangerous asthma attack or even a heart attack.

Steven sometimes came to my office for help. We'd run tests to check his heart and lungs, and then we'd reassure him that he was okay. This pattern went on for several years. And once he got his reassurance, he was back out there teaching Pilates and running and doing his usual thing.

During this time, Steven also experienced some difficult circumstances in his personal life. His son, whom he loved dearly, suddenly moved across the country to be with a woman he'd met on the Internet, effectively removing himself from Steven's life. Steven had an on-again, off-again relationship with his spouse. He had a strong sense of abandonment and was deeply affected when those he cared for seemed to reject him.

Then his business ran into financial trouble during the recession, and his number of visits to my office increased. I began to ponder what the real issue was for Steven. I started to ask him about his feelings of anxiety. He acknowledged that he had a lot of fear. It was clear that those conditions were affecting his health.

We began to dig into his foundational belief system about himself and about life and death. As it turned out, he had a lot of feelings of insecurity left over from his childhood. He had grown up in a faith system that was dogmatic and punitive, and he continued to believe that his ultimate destiny would be in a bad place and that he could never be forgiven for the things he'd done.

Though my role was not to be Steven's counselor, I did recommend some books that I thought might open him up to the ideas of compassion and forgiveness. Steven then went out and met with a faith leader from the denomination in which he grew up, but he chose a person who was compassionate and committed to the teachings of unconditional love, forgiveness, and hope.

Years later, when Steven came into my office for a check-up, he had a new tattoo. This one was very subtle. It was symbolic of the fact that he was loved, he said, and he began to cry as he told me about it. He said he felt completely forgiven for his past mistakes and that he had begun to feel truly alive and present for the first time in his life.

The most astonishing thing about Steven's story is that all the things he feared then actually came to pass. His son died of a drug overdose. His wife left him permanently. When he came in to see me after those things had happened, he was grieving and depressed.

"Do you need medicine for anxiety?" I asked him.

He shook his head. "No," he said. "I don't."

The old Steven surely would have been wrecked by these events, but this new Steven was resilient. He said that he didn't feel abandoned; even as his worst fears came true, he was able to remember that he was loved. "I'm not afraid," he said.

But that's not the end of the story. A while after that, Steven came in to see me with severe chest pain. He'd just had shoulder surgery, but the pain didn't seem to be the result of that. So I ordered some tests. It turned out that the bones of his spine, his scapula, and his ribs were riddled with tumors.

He was treated for the cancer, and for a while he went into remission. I saw him periodically over those years as he tried to fight off the disease. And even through this horrific period, his outlook remained positive. "I lived all those years healthy but afraid," he told me. "Which means that, really, I was unhealthy. Now, here I am. I've lost the people closest to me. I'm dying of this incurable disease. And yet every day, I'm alive and I'm well—and I'm not afraid."

Steven had gotten one more tattoo. Its essential meaning was that perfect love casts out fear. He no longer had panic attacks or palpitations; he had left all that behind.

When the cancer finally took him, he went without fear.

DON'T STOP HERE

Your life—the years ahead—belong entirely to you. No one can take them from you. Don't let any limiting belief keep you from claiming your life.

Remember that you do not need to spend money on some new gadget or health fad to have what you need to regain your health and to engage in your life's purpose. Over these 300-odd pages, you've absorbed a lot of information spanning the areas of health, spirituality, physiology, and even neuroscience. There are many great additional resources for you to continue exploring the areas that are most useful and inspiring to you. I know that the sheer number of different resources can be dizzying—but try not to become overwhelmed. Instead, pick one resource at a time, dig into it, and be patient with yourself.

The point is not to arrive at a specific destination. Rather, the point is to make this journey of increasing your competency in all the areas that encompass genuine health. So embrace the journey. Savor it. Don't rush.

If you deeply desire to be healthy, you will surely succeed. Start today, never stop, and don't let any negative voices—from yourself or from others—keep you from it.

ADDITIONAL RESOURCES
- *The Compound Effect* by Darren Hardy

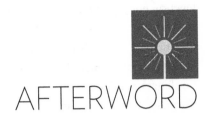

AFTERWORD

EARLIER IN THIS BOOK, I mentioned that my journey into meditation began and grew during a stressful time in my life as a young professional. It's interesting how life happens. Due to unforeseen changes in the healthcare marketplace, I went through a similar experience shortly after I began writing this book.

My medical practice had recently begun a series of expansions to improve community health and access to care. Then, at the same time, we experienced significant issues in cash flow due to the third-party payer system. I found myself once again working much harder and putting in longer hours than I had anticipated, at the same time seeing less economic reward for my work. My business had to borrow money if we were to keep trying to build and expand. We continually needed to devise creative solutions to keep things running smoothly and effectively.

During this time, I found myself having to miss a family vacation and working six clinics a week while also trying to write a book and maintain my role as leader of our healthcare organization.

This was a very stressful period, and I had to examine all of my habits. I was already a good sleeper, but I became a better one. Not only did I maintain my regular meditation practice and remain anchored in my foundational spiritual beliefs, but I dug more deeply into those beliefs and integrated them fully into my daily life. I ate healthy foods. I exercised as much as I could. My family was also fully supportive through this, and I'm deeply thankful to them for that.

The result was that I was able to maintain a positive mindset and a high level of energy, even as I began working at a pace I'd never known before. Indeed, the process of writing this book and dwelling in all of its principles helped me to thrive during this otherwise difficult time. I can say with complete confidence that the foundational messages and guidelines in this book gave me the health, the energy, and the positive outlook to pursue my purpose, even in the face of major obstacles.

I wish for the very same for you—and I believe that you're already on the path to get there.

What's more, I would love to have your feedback about how these resources have worked for you in practice. In order to develop a community of those of us who are engaged in this work, I've started an organization called Health Shepherds. Its founding concept is that we're all shepherding each other on this journey.

Thanks to the process of gathering the information in this book, I've come across many people who are involved in the same type of thinking and who are pursuing the same type of results. It's powerful and deeply encouraging to be part of this growing community that's dedicated to the pursuit of health and to our highest purpose. Health Shepherds is a place for all of us to engage together.

There's only one caveat: Health Shepherds is all about what we *can* do—not about what we can't do. It's a place where we can talk to each other about nutrition, movement, spirituality, purpose, and positivity. You'll find it at healthshepherds.com and at Facebook.com/healthshepherds. This is a place for positive discussions about resources that will help all of us on our journeys to our best selves. It is not a forum for negative comments about the larger systems that try to manipulate our thinking and habits. We are focused on shepherding each other to abundant pastures, not just pointing out the wolves, because we agree that negative focus escalates fear.

The more you know the truth, the less power the untruths will have over you. Light doesn't just penetrate darkness, it eliminates it. Let's focus on lighting the way for each other.

I invite you to join us.

ABOUT THE AUTHOR

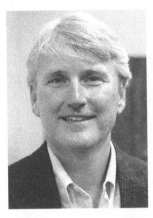

DR. GUS VICKERY is the founder and directing physician of Vickery Family Medicine in Asheville, North Carolina. He established his practice with a commitment to delivering holistic, compassionate, and evidence-based care. But when he realized that many of his patients were suffering from a complicated set of symptoms that were the result of underlying habits and could not be treated with conventional medical approaches, Dr. Vickery set out to develop a comprehensive program for treating his patients' ailments so that they could finally feel the good health and vitality that all of us deserve.

Dr. Vickery is a board-certified family physician and a graduate of the Medical College of Georgia. He was an honor medical student and received a scholarship and awards during his medical training. Dr. Vickery participates in teaching medical students and family medicine residents from The University of North Carolina at Chapel Hill medical school and East Carolina University medical school. Dr. Vickery has served as president of the Western Carolina Medical Society and as chairperson for Moving Healthcare Upstream, an initiative of the local Development Council. In 2005, Dr. Vickery founded Vickery Family Medicine, which has grown to 11 medical providers serving in three locations, including The Clinic at Biltmore, an innovative direct-to-employer clinic for The Biltmore Company. Vickery Family Medicine has received numerous awards for customer service and quality.

In addition to practicing full-time traditional family medicine, Dr. Vickery has spent countless hours studying cognitive behavioral science, motivational interviewing, neuroplasticity and brain training, meditation, biomechanical health and movement, nutrition, and the science of sleep. Dr. Vickery's holistic health curriculum has been used very successfully by The Biltmore Company for its Healthstyles initiative, a health improvement program for its employees. Dr. Vickery also studied health care delivery and founded Synergy Health Solutions, an innovative direct-to-consumer organization helping improve access and reduce cost while providing effective care.

Dr. Vickery remains passionate and committed to doing whatever is necessary to advance the cause of equipping everyone with the resources needed to experience his or her best health.

When not attending to his professional responsibilities, Dr. Gus Vickery spends his time with his best friend and wife, Kelle, and their three children exploring the outdoor spaces of Asheville, North Carolina.

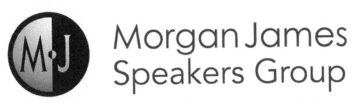

Morgan James
Speakers Group

www.TheMorganJamesSpeakersGroup.com

We connect Morgan James published authors with live and online events and audiences who will benefit from their expertise.

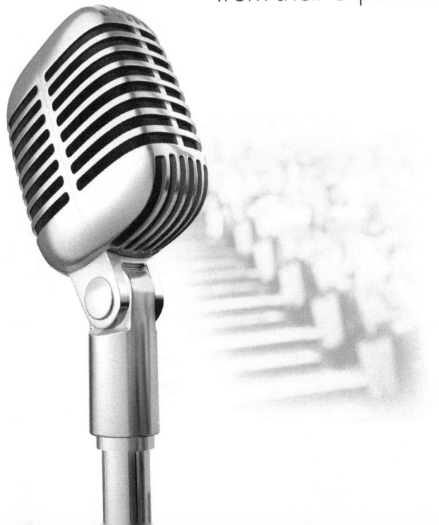

 Morgan James makes all of our titles available through the Library for All Charity Organization.

www.LibraryForAll.org